MW00805994

Praise for *Getting to Baby*

"Angela and Judy have not only masterfully summarized over a decade of scientific literature on the relation between diet and fertility, but also drawn on their invaluable clinical experience helping couples facing difficulties conceiving, resulting in a book that manages to convey complex information in an accurate but also relatable and compassionate way. Their unique professional relationship is evident in every page. Only the two of them could have written this fantastic book."

—Jorge E. Chavarro, MD, ScD, coauthor of *The Fertility Diet* and professor of nutrition, epidemiology, and medicine at Harvard T.H. Chan School of Public Health and Harvard Medical School

"For a plant-forward, evidence-backed guide on fertility nutrition, read *Getting to Baby*. Packed with helpful dietary tips and an introduction to intuitive eating, the authors encourage people of all body sizes to focus on supporting their health rather than weight loss when trying to conceive."

—Rachelle LaCroix Mallik, MA, RDN, creator of the Fertility Foundations nutrition course and founder of The Food Therapist, LLC

"I can't tell you how happy I was to read Dr. Angela Thyer and Judy Simon's new book *Getting to Baby*. They call it a 'food first' book . I would call it a 'you first' book. Too often my patients are sold books that focus on restrictive diets or—even worse—expensive supplements. In Angela and Judy's wonderful book they make sure to cover all the parts of a healthy lifestyle, including restorative sleep and moderate exercise. Diet is, of course, important and this book, full of healthy recipes and sensible plans to incorporate them into your lifestyle, focuses not on what we shouldn't eat but the delicious foods we need more of. Angela and Judy help us understand the basic science behind our choices and shine a light on today's headline issues like the new data on artificial sweeteners and our growing understanding of the microbiome. I wish I had this resource in medical school so my thousands of patients over the decades could have this book in their kitchen and this power in their hands."

—John McHugh, MD, FACOG, FACLM, founding leader of the American College of Lifestyle Medicine's Women's Health Group

"*Getting to Baby*, coauthored by two seasoned professionals in the field of female fertility, is an absolute gem for anyone embarking on the journey to parenthood. With decades of expertise and a heartfelt narrative of a special friendship, the authors provide a nourishing perspective on the intersection of food, lifestyle, and fertility. This book provides practical, real-world advice on how to incorporate specific nutrients, vitamins, and minerals that are essential for fertility into everyday life. *Getting to Baby* offers valuable strategies for all people, including those suffering from PCOS, to increase their odds of conception with a 'food-first' path toward the wonderful gift of pregnancy."

—Angela Grassi, MS, RDN, coauthor of *The PCOS Workbook: Your Guide to Complete Physical and Emotional Health*

"Judy Simon and Angela Thyer have created a wonderful book based on up-to-date nutrition science, a shared love of food, and real-world experience helping women conceive through their clinical practices and Food for Fertility classes. Not only are both authors skilled, experienced clinicians, but they truly care for their patients, and that shines through in this book. As a dietitian, I also appreciate that they include helpful cooking tips, recipe modifications, and advice for cooking on a budget to make their book accessible to as many people as possible. This book is much needed!"

—Carrie Dennett, MPH, RDN, author of *Healthy for Your Life*

"Dr. Angela Thyer and dietitian Judy Simon have written a must-read book for anyone considering pregnancy AND food as medicine . . . Use this as a guide and learn from experience."

—Bisi Alli, DO, FACP, dipABLM, member of the board of directors for the American Medical Women's Association

"If you're looking for fertility-friendly advice on nutrition with an evidence-based approach, look no further because you've found *Getting to Baby*. I am thrilled to have this resource to recommend to my patients who ask about optimizing their food choices for their reproductive health."

—Lora Shahine, MD, FACOG, reproductive endocrinologist and author of *Not Broken: An Approachable Guide to Miscarriage and Recurrent Pregnancy Loss*

"*Getting to Baby* is a delightful and inspiring read for anyone who is contemplating a pregnancy or has struggled getting pregnant. It will captivate your heart through moving stories of women who achieved a pregnancy after learning about the relationship between food and fertility. The authors gracefully blend evidence-based lifestyle recommendations with a practical guide of how to implement those recommendations into your daily life to improve fertility and overall health."

—Nancy Eriksen, MD, ACLM, coeditor of
Improving Women's Health Across the Lifespan

"I recently had the honor of reading *Getting to Baby* and I must say it's a remarkable resource for anyone looking to understand the connection between nutrition and fertility. Dr. Thyer's and Judy's expertise shines through as they make complex concepts accessible to all readers. Their dedication to empowering individuals to take control of their reproductive health through nutrition is inspiring and invaluable. The book delves into the science behind nutrition and its impact on fertility. It provides practical advice and dietary recommendations that can impact one's reproductive health, for both women and men. Their compassionate and empathetic approach to addressing the emotional aspects of infertility is commendable, offering a holistic perspective on the journey to conception. As a physician myself, I appreciate the evidence-based approach taken by Dr. Thyer and Judy, ensuring that readers receive accurate and up-to-date information. This book can also serve as a valuable resource for healthcare professionals looking to enhance their knowledge in this vital field. In a world where infertility affects so many, *Getting to Baby* is a beacon of hope and knowledge. I highly recommend this book to anyone seeking a holistic and uplifting guide on their path to parenthood."

—Paul C. Lin, MD, co-founder,
Seattle Reproductive Medicine

"This is not a diet book. Angela and Judy present a comprehensive and accessible plan to incorporate more plants into one's daily routine. As a fertility acupuncturist, I support people trying to conceive on their own or alongside assisted reproductive treatments. Questions about food frequently come up—what should I eat? Gluten is bad, right? What about meat? This book helps cut through the sea of conflicting advice and discerns science-based, clinically proven ways to support one's fertility with nutritious foods. I look forward to sharing this book. It can be a companion at the grocery store, helping you select delicious foods rich in nutrients. It's also your kitchen buddy inviting you to create dishes to savor and nourish."

—Lee Hullender Rubin, DAoM, LAc, fertility acupuncturist
and clinical researcher at Rosefinch Health

"As an obstetrician, I am so excited to find a book that connects the impact of diet on conception and pregnancy. Part cookbook, this guide makes eating healthy both simple and delicious while providing the science behind why it matters in your fertility journey. Be prepared to shake up your culinary world and come out the healthier for it!"

—Judy Kimelman, MD, obstetrician and gynecologist

"Angela and Judy have distilled their years of clinical and culinary wisdom into a book filled with practical, supportive guidance. It's an essential read for anyone wanting to take a food-first approach to fertility!"

—Kayli Anderson, MS, RDN, DipACLM, FACLM, lead faculty of the American College of Lifestyle Medicine's "Food as Medicine" course and creator of PlantBasedMavens.com

"Angela and Judy have done an incredible job distilling down the science from hundreds of academic studies and translating this into simple and practical advice for couples trying to conceive. *Getting to Baby* is a terrific guide to optimizing preconception health in men and women."

—Audrey Gaskins, ScD, associate professor of epidemiology at Emory Univerisity's Rollins School of Public Health

"As a registered dietitian who cares for couples dealing with fertility challenges, I so appreciate Judy and Angela's well-researched, food-first approach to optimizing diet and lifestyle for fertility. People struggling to conceive are exposed to a lot of information on diet, lifestyle, and dietary supplements, much of which is not science-based or makes unsubstantiated claims suggesting individual foods or supplements are the answer. *Getting to Baby* makes it clear it's the synergy of the overall dietary pattern, regular physical activity, and sensible supplementation that matters. They also highlight how these same strategies that can boost fertility in both women and men may reduce the risk of a number of common chronic health problems later in life. Their no-nonsense advice to commit some time each week to meal planning and preparation, physical activity, and other aspects of self-care make the information, and tasty recipes, great advice through fertility treatment and beyond! Health professionals will also appreciate this well-researched resource to educate their patients—and themselves—on science-based strategies to improve overall health and fertility."

—Hillary Wright, MEd, RDN, LDN, director of nutrition at the Wellness Center at Boston IVF

"The food-first fertility plan in *Getting to Baby* provides a patient-centered, health- and healing-orientated, scientifically sound approach that places attention on the whole person. It provides support and balance to complement technology-driven, conventional medical evaluation and treatment of infertility. I plan to enthusiastically recommend it as a resource to all my patients trying to conceive."

—Paula Amato, MD, MCR, professor of obstetrics and gynecology
and director of reproductive endocrinology and infertility
at Oregon Health & Science University

Getting to Baby

Getting to Baby

A Food-First Fertility Plan to Improve Your Odds and Shorten Your Time to Pregnancy

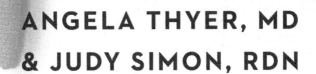

ANGELA THYER, MD
& JUDY SIMON, RDN

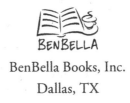

BenBella Books, Inc.
Dallas, TX

This book is for informational purposes only. It is not intended to serve as a substitute for professional medical advice. The author and publisher specifically disclaim any and all liability arising directly or indirectly from the use of any information contained in this book. A health care professional should be consulted regarding your specific medical situation. Any product mentioned in this book does not imply endorsement of that product by the author or publisher.

Stories and quotes have been graciously shared with permission of our clients.

Getting to Baby copyright © 2024 by Angela Thyer and Judy Simon

All rights reserved. No part of this book may be used or reproduced in any manner whatsoever without written permission of the publisher, except in the case of brief quotations embodied in critical articles or reviews.

BenBella Books, Inc.
10440 N. Central Expressway
Suite 800
Dallas, TX 75231
benbellabooks.com
Send feedback to feedback@benbellabooks.com

BenBella is a federally registered trademark.

Printed in the United States of America
10 9 8 7 6 5 4 3 2 1

Library of Congress Control Number: 2023039795
ISBN (trade paperback) 9781637744482
ISBN (electronic) 9781637744499

Editing by Leah Wilson and Rachel Phares
Copyediting by Elizabeth Degenhard
Proofreading by Denise Pangia and Cape Cod Compositors, Inc.
Indexing by WordCo Indexing Services
Text design and composition by Jordan Kolouch
Cover design by Sarah Avinger
Cover image © Adobe Stock / misskaterina
Printed by Lake Book Manufacturing

Special discounts for bulk sales are available.
Please contact bulkorders@benbellabooks.com.

This book is dedicated to everyone
who is ready to create new life in the kitchen.

Contents

Real-Life Testimonials

From participants in Judy and Angela's Food for Fertility class

"My outlook is wildly more positive. The class was an integral part of my finally achieving a healthy and successful pregnancy, which changed my life."

"You gave me permission to think in terms of being healthy rather than feeling like I should be denying myself and punishing myself to lose weight. It was a balanced approach to being healthy."

"I thought I would have to cut out so many foods; instead, I was introduced to so many new foods!"

"I feel like I have some control in this crazy IVF process in which I have little control. My diet is the one thing I can modify and control."

"Your program did it again. Pregnant with number two!"

"I loved all the new ideas to incorporate healthy eating. The process made it seem less daunting and manageable with a busy lifestyle. I loved the passion Judy and Angela have around food and promoting healthy lifestyles and pregnancies."

"I learned about the importance of meal planning and prepping ahead of time. One key habit that I have learned is to take one day out of my weekend to grocery shop and prepare food for the week. I'm more likely to eat healthy if I know exactly what's for dinner."

"The flavors were amazing! A lot of the vegetables were brand new to me and I am so excited to use them more. Leftovers became great for other meals. We used a leftover squash filling for breakfast with a fried egg on top."

"My husband had some sideways swimming sperm, so we applied the learnings you taught us about male fertility. He ate a lot of kale, spinach, anthocyanin-containing berries, beans, nuts, zinc-containing oysters, walnuts, and more, and improved his semen analysis. After three months, we conceived naturally without IUI."

"Thanks to you teaching me delicious ways to eat tofu and beans, I was able to eat them consistently, which made a big difference toward balancing my hormones to improve my fertility. We were able to conceive naturally without intervention, which surprised us."

"I feel so much healthier! I appreciate knowing that this isn't a diet, rather a lifestyle change, and that there are no off-limit foods. Your program helped teach me to make smart decisions about what—and how much—I put in my body."

"I really enjoyed trying so many new whole grains such as farro, forbidden rice, and quinoa. With these changes my glucose levels went from pre-diabetic range to normal."

"The goal 'we are going to eat salmon three times a week' was more helpful than 'eat more fish.' SMART goals made it more actionable. Making the time to set goals was helpful."

"I incorporated weightlifting per your suggestion to lower insulin resistance, and it helped a lot."

"I think the biggest change I noticed was feeling like I was doing things for a reason. There was a purpose to the meals."

"I liked all the additional ideas for integrating more nutritious foods into my diet. Learning why things are beneficial toward a healthy lifestyle and pregnancy means more than someone just telling you to eat more kale."

"The class gave me hope. It improved my relationship with my husband, not only because we could see improvements in my health, but because he enjoys the food, too. We are in a better place than when we were struggling with failed IVF cycles before taking this class."

"I'm more positive with going into IUIs knowing I'm preparing my body, and I feel confident in my food choices."

"I believe my pregnancy would have been much harder if I had not gotten healthy before getting pregnant. I had no issues with blood sugar and was able to stop taking metformin by thirty weeks."

"After the class, I no longer look at foods as being 'bad' or 'good.' I just think rationally and if I eat a hamburger one night for dinner, I'll skip the fries and try and take the dogs for a walk later."

"My outlook is a lot more positive. For the first time, I feel like I have control over my eating and my health. It's not one of those fad diets; it's thinking about what food you're eating and how it's affecting your health."

"I know this class has had an immense impact on my life and fertility."

Introduction

Welcome to *Getting to Baby*, the proven food-first plan to supercharge your fertility and shorten your time to pregnancy. No matter where you are in your fertility journey, whether you're just starting out, you've been at it for a while, or you've already begun fertility treatments and want to maximize your odds of success with in vitro fertilization (IVF), this book is for you. Our Food-First Fertility Plan has empowered thousands of people to change their mindset around food and health, fundamentally improve their physical and mental well-being, influence their embryo quality, and ultimately support healthy pregnancies. We've seen it. And studies prove it. Our plan will provide the solid, evidence-based guidance you are looking for.

Fertility treatments work best when you are in a state of optimal health, and food serves as the foundation for health. By eating well, not only will you enhance your fertility, but you'll improve your health overall. Although there is a wealth of research supporting the powerful connection between food, lifestyle, and fertility, most infertility specialists do not fully appreciate this connection, nor is it a significant part of mainstream fertility advice. Many physicians, too, have not received nutrition education in their training and may neglect to emphasize it as a vital part of your formula for success. With this book, we are excited to bring this valuable information to you to support your health and fertility!

So, what exactly is our Food-First Fertility Plan? It's a simple and accessible program that teaches you which foods help the most when you are trying to conceive and guides you in changing your diet to effectively incorporate them. We have guided thousands of patients through this program, and now we've distilled it into the pages of this book. In the chapters ahead, we are going to share which foods best support fertility and tell you which parts of the reproductive process they are able to influence. We'll tell you which foods could be reducing your fertility potential and suggest ways to lessen their influence. We'll give you practical approaches to changing your diet, and we'll provide recipes* and culinary tips to support any changes you need to make. *Getting to Baby* is a master class that lets you take advantage of the Food-First Fertility Plan at home. We'll guide you through the program and help you create actionable goals so you can see real results.

Throughout the book, you'll be hearing from some of our prior class participants so you can learn from their struggles and success: Olivia, who has irregular menstrual cycles and polycystic ovary syndrome (PCOS). April, who eats "clean" and exercises an hour a day but can't understand why she is not getting pregnant. Jodie, who is time-strapped and relies on convenience foods and fast foods. Revati, who had two failed IVF cycles and several miscarriages but isn't willing to give up. These are just a few of the women who adopted the Food-First Fertility Plan and are excited to share their stories with you. Although you may not have the same exact issues, you may find you have things in common with many women who are trying to get pregnant.

Now, a little bit about us. Dr. Angela Thyer, board certified in three subspecialties—obstetrics and gynecology, reproductive endocrinology and infertility, and lifestyle medicine—has taken care of patients for more than twenty years. She embraces holistic care, knowing how much diet, exercise, sleep, stress, and emotional support can strongly impact fertility—an approach that has allowed her to help thousands of women to realize their dream of starting a family. Angela is also uniquely qualified as a certified plant-based chef and

---

* For those with dietary needs or preferences, we've included labels as follows: V (vegan), VG (vegetarian), DF (dairy-free), and GF (gluten-free).

loves sharing her passion for culinary medicine and global cuisines. Judy Simon, an award-winning registered dietitian and health educator, has focused her practice on compassionately helping women and men nourish themselves to support their reproductive health. Judy promotes nutrition and fertility in a culturally sensitive, weight-neutral manner, and has shared her extensive knowledge by teaching and training graduate students, residents, and medical staff at the University of Washington and lecturing nationally.

It is rare for a subspecialist and a dietitian to work so closely together, but our partnership led to this amazing program to help women on their path to pregnancy. The two of us started working together due to our love of food and our common vision to help individuals improve their reproductive health. We came up with the idea for our class more than ten years ago with a common goal: to help women conceive by focusing on the foods that increase fertility while teaching them the skills in the kitchen to make cooking easy and fun. It sounds like such a simple thing, to focus on diet. Yet the power of food as medicine is frequently lost in the maze of complex fertility treatments. The existing research on how food affects fertility is overshadowed by supplements, pharmaceuticals, and IVF. No one is making a profit by promoting apples and broccoli. We know how much certain foods influence hormones and reproduction, and we created this program to help our patients more directly. Over the years, our program's success has grown; we've been invited to share our expertise with colleagues locally and nationally. Our patients and colleagues urged us to get this information out to an even wider audience so that anyone, at any stage in their fertility journey, can take advantage of this valuable knowledge. And now, we're thrilled to bring this program home to you.

The Food-First Fertility Plan can help everyone, because it is not a diet. People do not need to follow a rigid set of food rules—instead, they learn to intuitively nourish their bodies and become competent eaters. Every person comes to us and our program from a unique place, yet their end goal is the same: to have a baby. Our plan will shine a light and offer hope. When you are preparing for pregnancy and trying to conceive, your food choices matter, maybe more than anything else. We'll show you how to make eating for fertility simple and enjoyable and give you the tools to successfully adopt fertility-promoting habits to strengthen your reproductive health and help you achieve your dream of parenthood.

A Note on Language

We recognize that gender identity is fluid and that not everyone identifies on a binary scale. Our plan is inclusive for all. For ease in reference throughout the book, we have chosen to refer to individuals with ovaries or a uterus as women, and those who produce sperm as men, although this may not align with everyone's personal identifiers. We also acknowledge that many individuals, single or coupled, may be trying to conceive using donor sperm, donor eggs, donated embryos, or a gestational carrier. People build their families in a variety of ways including natural conception, assisted reproductive technologies, and traditional adoption. We have tried our best to use inclusive language and recognize that all paths to parenthood may be assisted by eating well and following a healthy lifestyle.

Chapter 1

The Fertility-Food Relationship

Test Your Knowledge

Eating pineapple can help women conceive.* True/False

My diet can impact how long it takes me to get pregnant.** True/False

What influences fertility?

There are some basic building blocks that you need for reproduction: an egg, a sperm, a fallopian tube, and a uterus. About once a month, ovulation occurs, with the release of an egg from the ovary. The window for an egg to be fertilized is typically less than twenty-four hours, but sperm can live for a number of days and still do their job. If sperm are in the vicinity at the time of ovulation, one lucky sperm may fertilize the egg just as it is getting picked up by the delicate fimbria of the fallopian tube. Over the next five days, hair-like projections inside the fallopian tube propel the fertilized egg

---

* True. Pineapple, along with a variety of other fruits and vegetables, is part of a plant-forward diet that will provide you with important nutrients to support your fertility.

** True. Get ready to learn how a plant-forward pescatarian diet can reduce inflammation, optimize your health, and reduce the time it can take to conceive.

down to the uterus. Once the embryo enters the uterus and lands on the lush uterine lining (called the endometrium), it may be drawn under the surface, allowing implantation to occur.

All the while, thousands of critical cell divisions—which are essential for the embryo to properly develop—are already occurring.

Infertility can occur if any of these steps are negatively impacted or interrupted—whether due to the quality of the embryo, the health of the uterine lining, or other issues with those other building blocks. The overall health of the body and external factors like toxins can also affect fertility.

The prevalence of infertility has been increasing over the past few decades. The World Health Organization (WHO) reports that infertility affects about one in six individuals worldwide, and, according to the Centers for Disease Control and Prevention (CDC), that number is closer to one in five in the United States. Why the increase? We can point to a couple of things. First, in the United States, people are having children later in life than ever before. Whether due to pursuing education and career goals first, putting off parenthood until they find a partner (maybe freezing their eggs, maybe not), opting to pursue solo parenthood later in life, or myriad other personal reasons, people are waiting longer to start their families. We frequently see women who are in their thirties or forties when they are trying for baby number one or two, and this comes with inherent challenges, because eggs lose quality as we age.

Second, our diets and lifestyles have changed dramatically in the past few decades, which has led to an increase in inflammation and insulin resistance. Processed foods and beverages currently make up over 60 percent of the average American diet and 50 percent of diets in other parts of the world. Red meat consumption has gone up as wealth has increased worldwide. Consumption of highly processed foods, combined with inadequate intake of vegetables, legumes, and whole grains, has led to increased prevalence of certain inflammation-related conditions like polycystic ovary syndrome (PCOS) and endometriosis, as well as reduced egg and sperm quality. Each of these conditions can negatively impact fertility. We're also more sedentary than ever. Many people have jobs that involve sitting in front of a computer and commuting by car, and we spend more of our leisure time on screens as well. This wreaks havoc on our metabolism.

Taken together, these conditions, worsening dietary patterns, and decreased physical activity have contributed to the dramatic increase in infertility worldwide.

Luckily, there are actionable steps you can take to increase your fertility. Our Food-First Fertility Plan is designed as the solution, to strengthen the health of eggs, sperm, fallopian tubes, and uterus by improving your body's metabolic health and decreasing inflammation.

As we go through this book, we will help you to understand which foods and activities can help you to accomplish these goals and support you in creating a plan that will work best for you. But first, let's take a deeper dive into how our diet can have a physiological impact on our fertility.

Does Weight Loss Help Fertility?

Women in larger bodies are frequently told by the medical establishment that losing weight will improve their chances of getting pregnant, but does it?

In a small study published in 2003, thirty-three women in larger bodies with PCOS went on a calorie-restricted diet. Polycystic ovary syndrome (PCOS) is a common condition affecting about 10 percent of women. Women with PCOS do not regularly ovulate (release an egg every month)—a problem if you want to get pregnant!—and generally have more insulin resistance than women without PCOS.[1] Twenty-five women in the study lost 5 percent of their body weight. Fifteen of those women resumed regular ovulation, and ten of the fifteen got pregnant naturally.[2]

But was the change due solely to weight loss, or perhaps better nutrition or more physical activity? Most likely, it was a combination. All three of these factors—weight loss, more fiber-rich foods, and exercise—reduce insulin resistance, which can help restart regular ovulation and therefore lead to higher natural conception rates in women with PCOS.

What about women who ovulate regularly and don't have PCOS? For women in larger bodies who ovulate regularly, studies have shown that weight loss does not typically improve pregnancy rates.

Rather than focusing on weight loss, we prefer to encourage everyone to focus on their health, because a nutrient-dense diet and regular physical activity can help everyone's chance of pregnancy. We discourage restrictive dieting while actively trying to conceive as it could deprive your body of necessary nutrients.

Anti-fat bias sometimes prevents people from getting the care they need and deserve. In 2021, the American Society of Reproductive Medicine published a committee opinion[3] that weight loss should not be recommended before offering fertility treatments, and no one's weight should preclude care (although some fertility centers have a BMI—body mass index—threshold for IVF). We recommend people of all sizes seek diagnostic testing and discuss treatment options with a fertility provider if attempts at home have been unsuccessful.

If you have PCOS and have heard that you should lose weight to help regain ovulation, know that there are alternatives that may help you to ovulate regularly that do not involve restrictive dieting. Plenty of women we have worked with have lowered their insulin resistance, reduced inflammation, and conceived by adopting our Food-First Fertility Plan without putting the focus on weight loss.

The Influence of Diet on Reproduction

The egg is the ultimate workhorse in the reproductive process. Sure, the sperm drops off its little bundle of DNA, which is an essential component of conception, but the egg provides not only its own DNA but also the meiotic spindle (responsible for lining up the chromosomes for cell division) and the mitochondria (the powerhouse, or energy reserve, of the cell) to facilitate cell division and early embryo development.

Egg health, then, plays a crucial role in fertility, and certain aspects of lifestyle such as diet, sedentary behavior, alcohol, tobacco, and toxins can impact an egg's health and assist or weaken the functions it performs.[4,5] Studies in mice, for instance, have shown that a high-fat/high-sugar diet can alter the distribution of mitochondria within the egg, alter their function and structure, and increase oxidative stress.[6] All of these disruptive changes can lead to cell damage, altered metabolism, and meiotic spindle instability. Ultimately, this damage may lead to real reproductive consequences such as fertilization failure, arrested embryo development, abnormal chromosome arrangements (aneuploidies), implantation failure, and miscarriage.[7]

Similar findings have been seen in human studies. In human volunteers, a high-fat, high-carbohydrate meal induced elevated oxidative and inflammatory markers in both normal weight and overweight subjects.[8] Women who follow the Food-First Fertility Plan eat more naturally occurring antioxidants and reduce inflammation in their bodies, reversing the metabolic changes that result from a Western-style diet. This may be why we see higher pregnancy rates in women of all sizes, occurring naturally or after IVF.

As eggs and their supporting cells age, oxidative stress can damage microcellular functions.[9] This damage accumulates over time[10] and can result in defective mitochondria that provide less energy for cell division within the egg once it is fertilized. (Accumulated oxidative damage also affects sperm, as healthy mitochondria are key to sperm's ability to move.) Some of this damage is part of normal aging, but some of it is due to additional oxidative stress from diet and lifestyle choices. By opting for certain diet and lifestyle habits, we can mitigate some of the cellular damage and enhance the chance of conception. *This is just one of the areas where the Food-First Fertility Plan can help.*

When it comes to optimizing egg health, the ninety days prior to an egg's release are the most important—when it is most vulnerable to external influences, positive or negative. It is during this time that the fluid-filled sac (follicle) and granulosa cells in the follicle begin to develop and prepare the egg. Anything the follicle is exposed to during that time can maximize or diminish the egg's potential for fertilization and normal cell division. So, every time an egg ovulates naturally, or when eggs are collected for IVF, the quality of those eggs has been influenced by their microenvironment during the past three months. The window of influence for sperm development is slightly shorter, about seventy days.

By taking care of yourself during these ninety days, you can best prepare your egg for fertilization. If you give your body what it needs from a nutrient standpoint, you'll make your best egg and best uterine lining. (Same goes for men—lifestyle choices over the preceding seventy days affect sperm health.) Certain foods can strengthen the health of your gametes, while other foods can increase oxidative damage and reduce their potential. Eating nutritious foods, getting physical activity, reducing your stress, sleeping well, and avoiding certain chemicals and substances that can harm fertility will all have a cumulative positive influence on your reproductive health.

The Research-Based Link Between Diet and Fertility

How do we know that diet has the power to influence whether someone becomes pregnant? A number of published studies have looked at what individuals recalled eating while they were trying to become pregnant.[11] One of the largest observational studies ever conducted, the Nurses' Health Study, followed a group of more than seventeen thousand women for eight years. Through yearly questionnaires, the investigators asked these women to report their pregnancies and miscarriages, as well as recall information about their diet, physical exercise, and smoking status. The initial findings were published by two of the main investigators, Jorge E. Chavarro and Walter C. Willett, in a scientific paper in 2007[12] followed by *The Fertility Diet* book in 2008.[13]

This observational study established the main advice for what we now know as the fertility diet. Among the more fertile group of women—the roughly 87 percent who conceived over the period of the study—researchers were able to condense their common diet and lifestyle habits into a list of takeaways that have become part of mainstream recommendations to support fertility. Having five or more of these lifestyle factors resulted in a lower chance of ovulatory infertility. This research got the medical world, for the first time, to acknowledge the link between lifestyle and fertility.

Here are the fertility-promoting habits researchers recommended as a result of the Nurses' Health Study:

- Avoid trans fats mainly found in ultra-processed and fast foods.
- Cook with monounsaturated fats like olive or canola oil.
- Consume protein from vegetable sources such as beans.
- Choose more whole grains.
- Consume full-fat yogurt or milk once a day.
- Take multivitamins with folic acid and B vitamins daily.
- Get iron from vegetable sources and supplements.
- Drink water and avoid sugary sodas.
- Lose a small amount of weight (5 to 10 percent) if menstrual cycles are irregular.
- Exercise thirty minutes or more daily.

Since the initial results came out from the Nurses' Health Study in 2007, researchers have been delving deeper into the effects of different dietary patterns on fertility. Studies on the Mediterranean diet, which consists of fruits and vegetables, whole grains, legumes, seafood, nuts and seeds, and olive oil, have shown the diet to be beneficial for natural conception[14] and for those couples undergoing IVF.[15] The Dutch dietary guidelines, very similar to the Mediterranean diet's with lots of fruits and vegetables, whole grains, legumes, eggs, fish, and nuts, have also been linked to increased chances of pregnancy for couples undergoing IVF.[16] There have been other studies that have specifically looked at how diet affects men's reproductive health and sperm, with the findings similar to those about women, showing that a diet rich in vegetables, fruits, whole grains, and fish helps to improve sperm parameters.[17]

Another well-designed but small study conducted between 2007 and 2017 looked at the combined effect of nutrition, lifestyle, and environmental factors on fertility. There were 357 women in a subgroup of the Environment and Reproductive Health (EARTH) study who were using IVF to achieve pregnancy. They all completed a food frequency questionnaire, where they were asked to share their dietary habits. The diet that proved to be the best for IVF outcomes emphasized fruits and vegetables, soy, and more seafood consumption over other animal proteins. They took additional folic acid, and those who were deficient in vitamin D and vitamin B12 took additional supplements. Women undergoing IVF whose diet most closely followed this fertility-promoting, or pro-fertility, pattern had the highest rates of pregnancy and the lowest rates of pregnancy loss. The authors state in their conclusion: "From a biological perspective, we hypothesize that there are many different pathways through which the 'pro-fertility' diet may be acting to promote fertility in women undergoing ART [Assisted Reproductive Technology] including enhancing the body's capability to synthesize, repair, and methylate DNA, suppress oxidative stress and support antioxidant defense, reduce systematic inflammation, and regulate glucose and insulin metabolism."[18]

We agree with the hypothesis drawn by the authors of the EARTH study: a diet that is anti-inflammatory and high in plants, soy, and seafood correlates with the highest fertility success.

Three Principles of a Fertility-Promoting Diet

Your diet fuels the building blocks of your reproductive system. It can combat harmful cellular changes due to inflammation and aging and allows for optimal embryo quality and implantation. The best diet for fertility follows common principles:

1. It is anti-inflammatory and high in fiber to promote a better uterine environment for implantation.

2. It is low glycemic to reduce inflammation and insulin resistance.
3. It is high in antioxidants to strengthen sperm and egg function.

As we've seen, there are a number of dietary patterns that follow these principles. It may be called whole food plant-based, plant-forward, pescatarian, or Mediterranean. We are going to refer to the pro-fertility dietary pattern as plant-forward most of the time, since these patterns emphasize foods from plants over foods from animal flesh. The core of these diets can be eaten over a lifetime. Many parts of the world follow similar eating patterns and healthy lifestyle principles including heritage diets from Africa, Asia, Latin America, and Native America. All these traditional heritage diets share commonalities, including a high number of fruits and vegetables, legumes, whole grains, and seafood. They minimize red meat, processed foods, and sugar. These are the principles of a diet for optimal reproductive health. Now let's take a look at each of these three principles and how they impact fertility.

Anti-Inflammatory, High Fiber

The fertility diet, the Mediterranean diet, the Dutch diet, and the EARTH study pro-fertility diet all share a foundation of fruits, vegetables, legumes, and whole grains. They emphasize plant sources of fiber, the inclusion of fish, and less red meat. And what is one basic component that makes plant foods so beneficial? If you said fiber, then you are correct. The benefit of fiber has been linked to our overall health, including our reproductive health. And of course, fiber works through the gut. When you think about reproduction and health, think about it starting in the gut where our food is digested.

Fiber and the Gut Microbiome

To understand the link between gut health and fertility, let's take a closer look at how our gut operates. Did you know that you coexist with more than thirty trillion microbes that live in your colon? These microbes are known as the gut microbiota and include bacteria, fungi, and viruses. Their environment, and the interface with the cells lining the wall of the colon, is called the gut microbiome. These terms are often used interchangeably, but the microbiota are the bugs themselves, whereas the gut microbiome describes how they function within their environment.

You and your microbiome are inexorably linked—at times, living in peaceful harmony, and at other times, in potential discord. The gut microbiome differs greatly from person to person. The foods you eat determine which species of microbes thrive in your colon and which ones die. How well you nourish your microbiome will influence your immune system, your hormones, your metabolic system, and your mood.

So how do you keep all those bacteria healthy? You may already know the answer: eat a wide variety of plants. Those bugs need their fiber! When you eat fiber, you're not using it for your own purpose. You can't. Only the microbes can digest it. Fiber gets passed through the small intestine to the colon where the microbes get to chow down. Fed bacteria are happy bacteria. More fiber leads to increased bacterial diversity, a higher total number of bacteria (they get to multiply), and a healthy gut environment.

The gut microbiome is, first and foremost, the key to maintaining immune health. A robust, diverse population of microbes leads to a thicker mucus barrier and more protection for the gut wall. The cells lining the gut are only one cell layer thick, and on the other side of that very thin interface are our immune cells in close communication. When you ingest animal proteins and ultra-processed foods, the microbes have nothing to digest (there's no fiber in these foods) and many die off. When the microbe population becomes out of balance, it is called dysbiosis. Dysbiosis can lead to the damage of junctions between cells in the wall of the colon, allowing for increased permeability, or leakiness. Increased permeability allows toxins and antigens to pass through the gut wall, where they can cause their own damage, or trigger activation of the immune system. When you are fighting off an invader in an acute setting, activating the immune system is a good thing. You want your immune system to be turned on. But if that very thin wall interface is not protected and the immune system is turned on all the time, it can result in chronic inflammation.

The cascade of events that flow from having chronic inflammation causes damage to our cells, tissues, and organ systems. Chronic inflammation is now recognized as the basis of many diseases, including some that cause infertility.

Fiber can help prevent these diseases by maintaining a healthy microbiome and preventing chronic inflammation. How does it do this? Fiber travels unchanged through the small bowel. In the large bowel, the bacteria break down fiber and transform it into small-chain fatty acids (SCFA). These signaling molecules are anti-inflammatory and anticarcinogenic, and modulate the immune response. They can even fix dysbiosis and a leaky gut wall. SCFA will promote the growth and diversity of good bacteria. Fiber and the SCFA are powerful! By eating a high-fiber diet consisting mainly of plants, the microbiome can better handle the intake of occasional foods without fiber and maintain a healthy ecosystem. So, if you eat a plant-forward diet most of the time, you can keep your gut microbiome harmoniously happy and occasionally enjoy a piece of salmon, chicken, or beef without causing it harm.

The Gut and Hormones

The influence of the gut doesn't end there. The gut microbiome is also quite involved with the endocrine system: scattered among mucosal and epithelial cells lining the gut are endocrine cells that secrete hormones. Dysbiosis can lead to the hormone estrogen "leaking" back into the bloodstream. Certain gynecological conditions such as PCOS and endometriosis are known to be "estrogen dominant" due to this higher amount of estrogen that has been reabsorbed into the circulation.[19] Modulation of the gut microbiota through food can positively (or negatively) influence these estrogen-dominant conditions.[20] Eating more fiber can lead to the repair of dysbiosis by shoring up the damaged gut wall, thereby reducing the inflammation involved in endometriosis and PCOS and curbing some of the resulting hormone dysregulation.

Women with PCOS demonstrate dysbiosis more frequently than women without PCOS, which may be influenced by an excess of androgens (other sex hormones).[21] It is unknown whether PCOS leads to dysbiosis or whether dysbiosis contributes to PCOS, or whether both are occurring independently.[22]

What we do know is that disruption of the gut-immune barrier can lead to activation of the immune system leading to chronic inflammation. Chronic inflammation can lead to dysfunction of the insulin receptor and insulin resistance, one of the hallmark signs of PCOS. Insulin resistance has been linked to elevated androgens, another common sign in PCOS, which can then lead back to dysbiosis.[23] Needless to say, it is quite a complex system that investigators are just beginning to understand. A plant-forward, whole-food diet, rich in fiber, can help heal the dysbiosis, break the cycle, and improve reproductive health.

A Low Glycemic Diet Promotes Fertility

The second principle of a fertility-promoting diet limits excess sugars and simple carbohydrates. Why? Excess sugars and simple carbohydrates spike your blood sugar, contribute to insulin resistance, and have an inflammatory effect on the body—all of which can inhibit fertility. When glucose levels in your bloodstream get too high, the mitochondria in cells can be overwhelmed by this energy excess and release free radicals, unstable molecules containing only one electron that are responsible for oxidative stress and tissue damage down to the level of our DNA.[24] Too much oxidative stress also contributes to generalized inflammation and insulin resistance.[25,26] This is the opposite of what you want, especially when you're on a fertility journey. When you are trying to conceive, you want your diet to be low glycemic so that your mitochondria have enough energy to do their job, but not so much that they are overwhelmed and set off a negative cascade of events.

A good way to control the level of glucose and resulting insulin in your bloodstream, in addition to limiting high-sugar foods themselves, relates back to fiber. Consuming foods that contain carbohydrates or sugars but *also* contain fiber can curb blood-sugar spikes. Fruit is a great example. A whole piece of fruit like an apple or orange contains sugar and fiber, while apple juice or orange juice is pure sugar without fiber. Whole grains like farro, brown rice, and whole wheat berries are carbohydrates that contain fiber; the processed and refined grains found in most bread or pasta have had the fiber removed.

Foods with fiber slow down gut transit, the rate at which glucose enters the bloodstream, thereby providing more stability for glucose and insulin metabolism. Ultra-processed foods, snack foods, and sugary beverages, including sweetened coffee and tea drinks, sodas, juices, and energy drinks, are typically low fiber and high glycemic. Women with PCOS may find a low glycemic diet especially beneficial, as they may be starting with higher insulin resistance.

Foods High in Antioxidants Are Key

The third and final principle of a pro-fertility diet is to eat plenty of high-antioxidant foods. Ultimately, one of the best things you can do to improve egg quality and function is to add more naturally occurring antioxidants to take on free radicals and reduce substances that increase oxidative stress. This is the crux of what we are talking about. Remember, as eggs and their supporting cells age, oxidative stress accumulates over time, which can result in cellular and DNA damage.[27] The same is true for sperm.

Increasing antioxidants (by eating plants) will curtail the risk of damage from oxidative stress and put egg and sperm in the best position to carry out the tasks they are responsible for, to the best of their ability. Shifting your diet toward fruits and vegetables also minimizes the risk of oxidative stress by bumping out some of the foods that can cause the stress in the first place (ultra-processed foods and excess sugars). It minimizes injury to the mitochondria within the egg and slows down the oxidative damage to the sperm.

Increasing antioxidants through food appears to be beneficial,[28] but antioxidants in the form of supplements offer only minimal additional benefit to women with infertility.[29,30] They may offer a negligible benefit for male subfertility. Results from studies that have looked at this connection are weakly positive, but data is poor quality.[31] Supplements are difficult to study since they are not regulated by the FDA like pharmaceuticals are. Even if there is biological plausibility for an antioxidant supplement like Coenzyme Q10 (CoQ10) to assist fertility, we simply don't have much solid data. The few well-designed studies that do exist are small, and any potential benefits of antioxidant supplements appear to be less than the benefits coming from the variety of antioxidants found in naturally occurring fruits and vegetables. Manufacturers of supplements are not able to claim any specific health benefits.

Supplements can also cause unintended consequences. Too much oxidative damage is bad, but antioxidants from supplements could swing the pendulum too far in the other direction. Some parts of our cellular development are extremely sensitive. At certain points in time, we benefit from the presence of reactive oxygen species, whereas other times they can be harmful. In the early stages of egg development, reactive oxygen species play a helpful role in the steroid pathway and hormone production. If that action is blocked by too much antioxidant activity, it is not in the egg's best interest. It is unlikely that one could have too much antioxidant activity from blueberries or spinach. Certain supplements are okay to take, but they should be specifically selected and used with care. We will discuss which supplements have the best evidence for use in chapter ten.

Our Food-First Fertility Plan

What's the proof that eating a plant-forward diet will help your fertility? We wish we had a perfectly designed, high-quality study where we randomized a group of couples trying to conceive to eat either a high-fiber, anti-inflammatory, low-glycemic, high-antioxidant diet, or a typical Western diet high in ultra-processed foods, sugar, and red meat, and then studied the pregnancy rates over the next year. This research would be great, but it doesn't exist, and it probably never will. Dietary studies are notoriously difficult to conduct, and people don't necessarily want to be placed in a randomized group. Dropout rates are extremely high for diet studies. And who's going to fund it? The cauliflower consortium? The chard council?

What we do have is our combined experience with thousands of individuals we have helped over the past twenty-plus years. These women, and some of their partners, made changes to their diet as we suggested in our Food-First Fertility Plan and discovered success that had previously eluded them. They got pregnant naturally when they didn't think they could, or they made better quality embryos with their next IVF cycle and conceived with the help of technology. Most also incorporated more physical activity into their daily routine and embraced a healthier lifestyle—we'll get into all of this in the coming chapters. We want you to follow in their footsteps and achieve pregnancy sooner with this Food-First Fertility Plan.

The Challenge

We hope we have enlightened you that eating a high-fiber, low-glycemic, anti-inflammatory diet full of fruits, vegetables, whole grains, legumes, and fish is key to optimizing your fertility, but knowing facts on their own isn't enough. If you're like most people, there may be some things you'd like to do to improve your diet and focus it toward optimizing your reproductive health. You may be excited to incorporate some of these changes, but making changes is not so easy.

Dietary patterns are hard-wired for most of us. Eating is a repeated behavior. We do it every day, multiple times a day, and those patterns get ingrained. Most people choose what to eat based on taste, cost, convenience, and habit. If it's easy, and it's what you've been accustomed to, you usually go with the flow. Moving to a more plant-focused diet may take extra thought and planning, especially at the beginning, but we know you are up for the challenge. New habits are best established by making small changes over time. For most people, this means learning how to make vegetables and legumes that taste delicious and feel satisfying as a meal. The foods need to offer enough excitement and variety to your tastebuds to sustain the change. Once you've increased your culinary prowess and have developed a comfort level cooking globally inspired plant-based recipes, you'll be on your way to supercharging your fertility!

We'll show you how to make eating for fertility simple, easy, and enjoyable. Most of the recipes we've included take thirty to fifty minutes (real food takes time!) to prepare. From there, it is easy to modify them to suit your personal taste. Our plan encourages you to eat more vegetables and legumes, move more, and enjoy time with friends and family on your path to pregnancy. We encourage progress over perfection. This book is not meant to replace working one on one with a dietitian or reproductive endocrinologist, but it will hopefully give you a big jump start. Focusing on the foods you eat every day and the way you intentionally spend your time can benefit your health in multiple ways, not just when it comes to fertility.

In the first part of this book, we'll take you step by step through foods that may be unfamiliar to you. We'll share the specific fertility benefits for each of these food groups. By providing culinary tools and recipes, we'll help you to get more comfortable in the kitchen. We'll also ask you to set some weekly goals to incorporate new foods or new preparations.

Then, we'll share extra fertility lifestyle boosters you'll want to know about and show you fertility disruptors that you can avoid. Finally, we sum it up with a comprehensive six-week blueprint designed to help you incorporate changes over time with a slow and steady approach. We hope that these recommendations help you to optimize your fertility and ultimately achieve your goal of pregnancy.

Many times, a story is the best way to illustrate a concept. Seeing what another person has gone through and hearing about their struggles can shed light on obstacles that you may also be facing. So, throughout this book, prior participants of our program will warmly share their stories of triumph so you can see how they faced obstacles and were resilient in the face of adversity. Although it can feel isolating, infertility is a common diagnosis shared by millions of women across the globe. Narratives highlight these all-too-common experiences and frustrations women go through as they try to conceive and change their habits. Understanding that you are not alone is important to build your resilience.

Before we do any of that, however, let's talk about some concepts that will help you successfully adopt the Food-First Fertility Plan.

Chapter 2

Moving Toward a Food-First Fertility Plan

Test Your Knowledge

Changing a habit takes a lot of willpower. True/False

*Cooking meals from scratch can save time and money.** True/False

B efore we dive into talking about specific foods and their fertility benefits, we're going to introduce some tools to help you change your diet from whatever you may be currently eating to one that provides the most benefit to your fertility. A diet transition like this needs time to be successful. Your habits around food preferences are longstanding, and it's rare to be able to change them overnight. We all follow our routines and eat what we're used to; we enjoy our traditions and habits. So we want to set you up with some resources designed to help you change your mindset about food, diet,

---

* False. Changing a habit takes motivation, confidence, and planning. If you are well prepared, you are more likely to succeed, and you do not need to rely on willpower.

** True. Meal planning and home cooking actually save both time and money (and use better ingredients!). We will teach you strategies to prepare quick, delicious meals at home that you'll enjoy.

and lifestyle, and the tools to make this change accessible and fun. This will enable you to sustainably alter your eating habits at your own pace and with confidence, implementing the Food-First Fertility Plan in a way that works for you.

This plan will culminate in the fertility blueprint; over six weeks, you'll be able to successfully transition to a plant-forward pattern of eating to maximize your reproductive potential. But herein lies the challenge. You'll need to appeal to all the factors that influence what you choose to eat in the first place, including cost, convenience, and taste. We want to set you up for success, which is why we spend so much time expanding skills around plant-forward cooking. It's hard to get more plants into your diet if you don't know how to make a bunch of vegetables and beans taste delicious. In *Getting to Baby*, we include valuable culinary skills, tips, and recipes so you can get busy in the kitchen. Ideally, you want to make eating plant foods easy, flavorful, and satisfying to crowd out the less healthy options you may be used to eating. This is a basic tenet of behavioral science: make your ideal behavior the easier choice. Most of what we do, we do out of habit. Changing habits takes thoughtfulness, planning, intention, and time. It will include building your skills in the kitchen, broadening your palate to embrace new flavors, and establishing routines, all with a healthy dose of patience.

The Fertility Plate, a Visual Guide

We came up with the idea of the "Fertility Plate" as an easy tool to guide your meals and snacks. A rough estimate is that half the plate should be vegetables, about a quarter of the plate whole grains, and the last quarter of the plate protein from legumes, fish, or eggs. Healthy oils can be used for cooking or as part of a salad dressing. Extra foods to consider for the plate, or for snacks between meals, would include fruit, nuts, and seeds, and an optional serving of whole-fat dairy.

The Fertility Plate

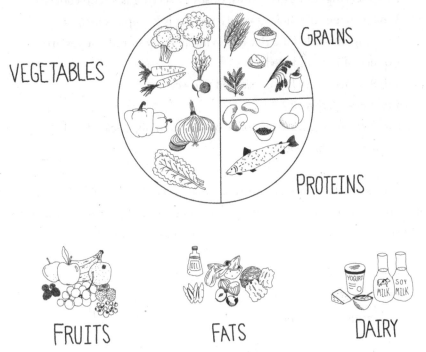

Illustrated by Ben Sanders

We think it is much easier to internalize this plan by visualizing the actual food on a plate (especially when half the plate should be veggies), but for those who prefer to have the daily/weekly recommendations laid out in numerical terms, this information can also be described as the number of servings of each food group you should target. The quantities you consume will vary day to day based on your activity level and personal preferences.

Here are the daily servings that comprise the Fertility Plate, including the recommended frequency and how each food group is helping to make the best sperm, eggs, and uterine lining:

5 to 6 servings of vegetables (1 serving is 2 cups of greens, or 1 cup of raw or 1/2 cup cooked vegetables)

2 to 3 servings of fruits (1 serving is the size of your fist)

1 to 3 servings of beans, lentils, or soy (1 serving is ½ cup cooked)

3 to 6 servings of whole grains (1 serving is ½ cup cooked)

1 serving of whole-fat dairy (1 serving is 1 cup of milk or yogurt)

1 ounce of nuts and seeds

6 to 9 ounces fatty fish or seafood per week

3 to 7 eggs per week

1 to 2 servings extra-virgin olive oil, avocado oil, or canola oil (1 serving is 1 tablespoon)

This is the food balance we're ultimately aiming for. We know it won't happen overnight, so we've designed our program to help you get there. Here are those tools, which we'll cover in the remainder of this chapter:

1. Your intrinsic motivation and confidence
2. SMART goals
3. Eating competence

Each of these components can make a huge difference in your ability to successfully and sustainably implement the Food-First Fertility Plan.

Identify Your Motivation and Increase Your Confidence

First things first. It's time to identify your *why*, your motivation to change. This is the primary key to your success. For most of you, getting to baby may be all the motivation you need. Linking a desire for change to an emotion or aspiration typically leads to greater success than knowledge alone. If your motivation does not incentivize you, no amount of information will be persuasive. On a scale of 1 to 10, with 10 being highly motivated, if you're at a 7 or greater, that's a good place to be.

In addition to internal motivation, you'll need the confidence that you can succeed in changing your habits over time. If you are motivated but lack confidence, you may allow obstacles to get in your way, especially when it comes to food choices. So let's use the same scale, 1 to 10. How confident are you right now that you will succeed in making changes? If you are starting at a 6 or less, that's okay. Our Food-First Plan is here to build up your confidence through the use of weekly goals and culinary skill-building. Visualizing the obstacles you may face in certain circumstances and planning a strategy to overcome them will lead to greater success. If, for example, there are no healthy foods available at work, you can pack carrot sticks and almonds for an afternoon snack so you don't end up wandering into the break room and grabbing chips!

For a behavior change to stick, you need to have both high motivation (the will) and high confidence (the skill). We want you to take the role of behavioral scientist in this process, to recognize that changing decades of ingrained habits is going to be challenging, but accepting that micro-wins on a daily basis will lead to larger gains over time. You only need to make a few small steps forward each week to make progress, and, over time, your confidence will grow. Strive for balance and take it slowly as you merge new health habits into well-worn and loved traditions. We are confident that you will continue to move toward your goal of family building. And your new plant-forward diet will serve you well for a very long time!

Setting SMART Goals

One of the best ways to establish a new habit is by setting goals for yourself that actually work for *you*. With that in mind, we've implemented the SMART framework for goal-setting. SMART is an acronym:

- Specific
- Measurable
- Achievable
- Realistic
- Timely

SMART goals work because they are small and attainable, which allows you to take away a win each week as you build toward your long-term objective, a diet that optimizes your fertility and moves you forward on your path to parenthood. Achieving your goals each week yields positive feelings, leading to more positive results, moving you in a winning feedback loop. These weekly accomplishments build self-efficacy and confidence. We find it is best to focus on the goals that *add* more nutritious foods to your diet rather than setting goals to limit certain foods. For instance, try overnight oats, add beans to a salad, or include a handful of spinach to a stew. These are all additions, and you'll be increasing the best foods for reproductive health and crowding out the others. You can do this at your own pace: many of our class participants actually worked on the same goals for weeks. Accountability also works wonders to establish new positive habits. You can be accountable to yourself, or you can share your goals with a friend or partner.

If we were meeting with you one on one, we would ask you to set new discrete goals each week. This is how you can make progress on your Food-First Fertility journey. These goals should be actual behaviors and tasks that you can carry out rather than a long-term objective. We'll suggest SMART goals at the end of each chapter, but we want you to make your own as well. Something like "I will buy curly kale this week for my Wednesday salad" works well, but "I want to lose ten pounds in two months" doesn't work. Weight loss is a common objective, but it is not a behavior you can change. Focus on very specific changes around food or lifestyle behaviors. Goal-setting should lead to small changes in behaviors that become habits. Those habits, over time, will make reaching your long-term objectives more likely. Making small changes in your food choices and cooking new recipes each week will lead to a noticeable shift in your dietary pattern over time.

To break a food habit, the opposite holds true: make it invisible, unattractive, difficult, and unsatisfying. How do you do this? Don't keep ultra-processed snack foods in your home, or if someone else in your household buys it, have them hide it. If it's not in your home, it's going to take effort to go out and buy it. That additional step of increased friction takes more energy to overcome, making the behavior less accessible.

Eating Competence

Sometimes eating feels rushed. Other times it can feel like a chore. Ideally, eating would involve a lovely, multi-course meal with some traditional dishes and some novel foods to try. You'd sit down with friends and family and take the time to enjoy the meal, filling your body with food that had been lovingly prepared with delicious flavors, aromas, tastes, and textures. You would eat to feel satisfied and to meet your body's nutritional needs. Being a competent eater[1] means you enjoy the pleasure of food and are curious and flexible trying new foods. You know enough about the nutritional content of foods to make choices that will meet your body's needs, and you have the skill to plan meals ahead of time rather than eating haphazardly. Lastly, you would listen to internal cues, eating until you are satisfied. Throughout our Food-First Fertility Plan, we'll talk about the ideas of external and internal competencies as they apply to your eating habits.

External Competencies: Culinary Medicine

External competencies have to do with your knowledge of the nutritional value of food, meal planning, and cooking skills. This knowledge ties directly to culinary medicine. Culinary medicine is a discipline that brings together nutrition and culinary skills to achieve our best state of health. Understanding that the foods you eat are as powerful as any prescription medicines, vitamins, or supplements you take lets you use that knowledge to influence your food choices.

Culinary medicine strives to introduce world flavors and different culinary plant-based traditions so you can eat deliciously and incorporate more whole foods into your diet. Of course, you want meals to taste great, not bland. Spices are secret ingredients to make your food more appealing. And your overall health will be elevated by learning these culinary skills. By shifting to a plant-forward diet with more fiber and nutrients, you will be able to reduce your insulin resistance and inflammation, improving your fertility.

We want you to feel comfortable in the kitchen so you can be creative and willing to explore new cuisines and recipes with nutrient-dense foods that taste delicious, too. That's why, in each of the food chapters, we share specific skills and recipes so you can gain confidence in the produce aisle, at the farmers market, and in your own kitchen. By gaining culinary skills so you can be an excellent home cook, planning meals and cooking will become easier and more efficient. Confidence in the kitchen will go a long way in your ability to be a competent eater and make intentional choices about what to buy and cook. Your dishes will have strong sensory appeal, so you can find great joy in sharing them, too.

Internal Competencies: Intuitive and Mindful Eating

Part of being a competent eater is being attuned to your body's signs of hunger and satiety and providing it with what it needs. It is important to eat regularly and provide your body with a consistent supply of energy to function optimally without skipping meals. That's why intuitive and mindful eating are part of developing your internal eating competence.

These tools involve slowing down and listening to your internal cues rather than external noise telling you what you should or shouldn't eat. Intuitive eating rejects the diet culture and restrictive eating patterns. It encourages eating for pleasure and nourishment. As you get comfortable with vegetables and legumes, you don't need to worry about limiting yourself. Eat until you are satisfied. (For a deeper dive into this concept, the book *Intuitive Eating* by Evelyn Tribole, MS, RDN, and Elyse Resch, MS, RDN, has been groundbreaking in getting people to think differently about their relationship with food. It is now in its fourth edition.)[2]

When you are eating to satisfy hunger, engage your senses. Most of us think about the taste and smell of food, but are you also appreciating the appearance of the food on the plate, the aroma, the sound of the crunch, and the textures of the food as you slowly chew? Do you appreciate the different tastes within the same meal (sweet, sour, salty, bitter, and umami)? Taking the time to consider the many complex flavors in your food will help you enjoy it more. When we share a meal and conversation with others, most of us slow down, which allows us to enjoy the meal more. Follow the same idea when you are eating by yourself—no screens, streaming, or scrolling. Practice eating mindfully and savor the flavors and textures as you chew your food. Slowing down the eating process allows time for the satiety signal to register in your brain, and you may find yourself eating less.

When moving toward a whole food diet, you may need to adjust to the taste of real foods that have not been industrially processed. Whole foods taste less intense than ultra-processed foods, which are designed to be hyperpalatable. It may take some time to unravel years of conditioning to the combinations of high-salt, sweet, and fat found in snack foods. But after about two weeks, you will begin to appreciate the flavors and textures of whole foods. The same is true if you are trying to reduce added sugars or artificial sweeteners. It will take some time, but as you wean off, you will become better able to appreciate the sweetness in whole fruits.

Even though we know that ultra-processed foods are not nutritious, we prefer not to call them bad or off limits. Doing so can lead to a sense of deprivation and a dysfunctional relationship with food. We recognize that most of us eat some foods or food-like items that offer very little from a nutritional standpoint. They can be ubiquitous in social situations and are associated with fun times with friends. It's okay. When you give yourself permission to eat or drink these foods on occasion, you may find you don't crave them as much. There is no need to be perfect. Be kind to yourself and practice self-compassion. Your primary role as an intuitive eater is to make sure you have honored your body's needs with gentle nutrition, not rigid rules.

Recognizing hunger and fullness sensations are an important principle of intuitive eating. To get in the practice of tuning in to your hunger and fullness signals, each time you sit down to eat a planned meal or snack, rate your hunger and fullness: On a scale of 1 to 10, how do you perceive your hunger? Extreme hunger is a 1, neutral is a 5, and extreme fullness is a 10. Ideally, you will feel most comfortable between a 3 and 7. Take inventory throughout the day to bring more awareness to your sense of satiety or fullness. Try never to get too hungry or too full. To help you keep track of your hunger and fullness, there are apps you can download to your phone, or you can jot down your hunger rating in a journal. This easy exercise takes just a second of pause before meals and snacks, but the benefits are far-reaching. Women have repeatedly told us that intuitive and mindful eating skills are some of the most valuable things they learned from our class.

Sometimes we eat when we are stressed, bored, or lonely. With the ups and downs of infertility, some women eat to feel comfort. Having a full belly does provide a sense of well-being, but eating when the body does not need it isn't helpful in the long run. If you find yourself eating in some of these situations, take a pause and rate your hunger. If you're not actually hungry, consider an alternative to eating. Walking outside and connecting with nature (rain or shine), taking a warm bath or shower, or texting a friend and arranging to talk later in the day can lift your mood and bring comfort in a different and equally satisfying way.

Women's bodies are remarkable in their gift to give life, and women of all sizes become pregnant and have healthy babies. If your doctor asks you about your weight, enlighten them with what you've learned, and what you're working on to improve your health like eating competently, moving more, and managing stress. Doctors don't know everything, and you might teach them something!

When Lifestyle Changes Aren't Enough

If you are just starting on your fertility journey, you may get pregnant right away, or it may take much longer. We encourage you to use the tools in this book to develop resilience. Many of the women we've worked with told us how fulfilling it was to fall back on the principles of eating well, getting regular exercise, and reducing stress to stay grounded throughout the process of trying to conceive.

It's important for you to know that there are some things that a healthy lifestyle cannot overcome, and for these conditions, we recommend you seek the assistance of a fertility specialist.[3] The reason is that the chance of pregnancy decreases over time.

At any age, the greatest percentage of pregnancies occur within the first six months of trying. The number of pregnancies significantly drops the second six months, and even more every year thereafter.

Many people delay making an appointment with a fertility specialist due to distractions, or fear of what they may discover, but there is nothing to be gained by delaying once you are ready to build your family. In fact, the delay can cause harm if years go by, since female age has the greatest effect on fertility rates. If pregnancy does not come easily, a medical issue may be contributing to the problem. Ask for basic testing and start treatments if recommended. Whether you are trying for baby number one or two, fertility clinics are there to provide medical services to help you achieve your family goal. And remember, you are in the driver's seat. Once you are given information and options, you will decide what is best for you.

Based on where you live, you may choose to seek the advice of an obstetrician gynecologist, primary care physician, naturopathic physician, advanced practice provider, acupuncturist, or Traditional Chinese Medicine (TCM) doctor, but the most advanced and detailed care will be available from a reproductive endocrinology and infertility (REI) doctor. Available in most major metropolitan areas, these subspecialists have completed four years of medical school (earning an MD or DO), four years of residency in obstetrics and gynecology, and an additional three-year fellowship in the subspecialty of reproductive endocrinology and infertility. REI physicians will be able to provide the full scope of advanced reproductive services, including IVF. The Society for Assisted Reproductive Technology website[4] lists member clinics that are committed to providing the highest standards of care.

Next Steps

Now you have the tools you'll need to start making changes. Near the end of this book, we'll give you a blueprint to help you go from your current diet to a pro-fertility one, along with some sample daily menus. But first, you're probably bursting with excitement to learn more about the actual foundation of the plan—the food! Let's start talking about the foods you'll want to incorporate into your diet to support your fertility.

Erin's Story

Judy met Erin when she was struggling to have a second baby. She had been through many prior miscarriages and two ectopic pregnancies, so she expected a rocky journey since having her first child had been so difficult. Erin and her partner tried to conceive naturally for more than six months without success. Erin worried because she was now over thirty-five and felt she was overweight. Her primary care provider implied that the residual baby weight from the first pregnancy was the problem, but her lab results were better than they had ever been. She returned to the fertility clinic where she had gone for help with her first successful pregnancy. This time she took her fertility doctor's advice and reached out for a nutrition consultation with Judy. She was happy she did.

From a food perspective, Erin always had obsessive ideas about nutrition: "I'd gone to Weight Watchers for ten years and I had internalized dieting messages." During her first pregnancy she had stuck to 100-calorie snack packs, which were often unsatisfying. In the past, she memorized the lowest calorie snacks. Now that she thinks of food from a fertility perspective, "I focus on the positive benefits of food rather than just the calories. I give myself permission to eat without guilt." Even when she is tired or busy, she feeds herself competently and truly enjoys the food she is eating.

Erin worked on accepting her body. She wanted to focus on nourishment rather than deprivation. So, she and Judy worked together to focus on her relationship with food. It immediately took the pressure off dieting, and she was able to focus on intuitive eating. "If I am hungry for almonds, I no longer count them. I enjoy a handful of almonds and if I need another handful, I will eat them, too." Erin worked to find a way to trust her body and was ready to try again to conceive. She had decided to try up to six rounds of intrauterine insemination (IUI) and, if not successful, she would consider IVF. She didn't enjoy the required medications, but was able to keep her focus on intuitive eating. She was thrilled to successfully conceive during her sixth IUI treatment and went on to deliver a heathy baby.

Chapter 3

Eat the Rainbow!

Test Your Knowledge

There are no pesticides on organic produce.* True/False

Fruit isn't healthy because it is too high in sugar.** True/False

Why are we so excited to talk about eating a rainbow of fruits and vegetables? Because each color in fruits and vegetables provides different essential phytonutrients to support your health and fertility. Plus, they are absolutely gorgeous and taste delicious! By reducing oxidative stress in the body, fruits and vegetables are the soldiers in the fight against inflammation. Inflammation, as we've learned, may contribute to infertility and other chronic diseases. The higher the content

---

* False. Organic farmers use pesticides and herbicides from a regulated list from the Environmental Protection Agency (EPA). They use them after other preventative measures have been taken. Fortunately, EPA regularly samples conventional and organic produce and more than 99 percent were within safe limits and more than half had no detectable pesticide residue. Wash all produce under running water before consuming.

** False. What better way to enjoy sweet flavors than from fruit? Eating the whole fruit will provide you with fiber, vitamins, minerals, antioxidants, and flavor. Much of the sugar from fruit is actually in the form of fructose, which has a relatively mild impact on blood glucose and insulin levels.

of fruits and vegetables in the diet, the stronger your anti-inflammatory benefit.[1]

The number and variety of fruits and vegetables out there is vast, and each has a different taste and texture. They contain lots of fiber and are low in saturated fat. You can prepare them in a multitude of ways: raw, steamed, roasted, grilled, seasoned, marinated—the list is long! But whether cooked or raw, they will become a base for your meals in our Food-First Fertility Plan.

Fruits and vegetables consist mainly of carbohydrates, which provide most of the energy for us to function. They contain some protein and fat as well. Most plants fall into the category of complex carbohydrates, meaning they can be broken down into glucose for immediate energy use or stored as glycogen for later. Complex carbohydrates should make up most of one's daily intake, ideally providing 40 to 70 percent of our daily energy.

Health Benefits

Fruits and vegetables are major sources of fiber, which, as we know, is the best and only food for your microbiome. Gut bugs love plant-based fiber, so one way to increase the growth and diversity of gut bugs is to eat more vegetables. Variety and numbers matter—think about each color group as feeding different species of bacteria (more on the specific benefits of each color of the rainbow in a minute). The polyphenols from colorful vegetables are fabulous for the microbiome. When you focus on improving your gut microbiome, you are indirectly helping your body support its reproductive function.

The average woman in the United States only takes in about 15 grams of fiber per day. The Dietary Reference Intake (DRI) recommends at least 25 grams of fiber daily, but for optimal fertility, we recommend an even higher level, around 40 grams per day. See the fiber charts we've included: Did you know that raspberries are a fiber powerhouse? How about broccoli and peas? (Okay, peas are actually a legume, so of course they're going to have more fiber.)

Vegetable	Total Fiber (grams per serving)
Broccoli	5.0
Brussels sprouts	4.0
Carrots	3.0
Cauliflower	2.0
Corn	3.5
Peas	9.0
Romaine lettuce	2.7
Sweet potato	3.0

Fruit	Total Fiber (grams per serving)
Apple	4.5
Banana	3.0
Blueberries	2.0
Orange	3.0
Pear	5.5
Raspberries	8.0
Strawberries	2.0

Fruits and vegetables create fullness due to the fiber. You can pretty much eat as much as you want (as long as they're not deep fried)! The fiber in plants takes up space but provides no calories. We can teach our tastebuds to bask in the flavors of colorful fruits and vegetables and eat to our heart's content, rather than tiptoeing around the endless parade of fake foods and feeling like we can't eat too many.

It's no coincidence that Americans fall short on getting their recommended fiber intake because they fall short on getting the recommended number of fruits and vegetables—the two deficiencies are related. According to the dietary guidelines for Americans, a minimum of five servings of fruits and vegetables are recommended daily,[2] but most people consume an average of two servings of vegetables and one serving of fruit per day.[3,4]

If five servings is the minimum recommendation, more must be better, right? Yes, in fact it is. Eating seven to eight servings of fruits and vegetables daily is highly protective, and can decrease the risk of certain cancers, cardio-vascular disease, and all cause mortality.[5,6] Studies have shown that around seven to eight servings of fruits and vegetables a day can boost your mood in the short term[7] and reduce your risk of chronic disease and death in the long term.[8] Eating more fruits and vegetables has also been correlated with decreased depression.[9] More fruits and vegetables have been associated with a greater sense of positivity, well-being, and happiness.[10] Who doesn't want to feel more curious, creative, and satisfied with life?

Eat Happy! Be Plant-Forward

A plant-forward diet is one that comes *mainly* from plants but is not the same as a vegetarian or vegan diet. Food from plants—fruits, vegetables, legumes, whole grains, nuts, and seeds—are embraced and celebrated, but food from animal sources can be included. In fact, an entirely plant-based diet will more frequently result in deficiencies in vitamin B12, iron, calcium, choline, iodine, and omega-3 fatty acids (DHA and EPA), which need to be treated, especially when trying to conceive. Eating plant-based at least 80 to 90 percent of the time can get you most of the health advantages, including improved reproductive health, better mood, and reduced risk of diabetes, heart disease, and certain cancers, while at the same time reducing your likelihood of developing nutritional deficiencies. So go ahead, call yourself a plant-forward eater!

Fertility Benefits

Vegetables and fruits are key to supercharging your fertility. Loaded with anti-oxidants, they are anti-inflammatory. Most vegetables (excluding potatoes) are also low glycemic. Whole fruits vary in their glycemic load, but that's okay because they come with their own fiber to slow down glucose absorption. Fruits with lower glycemic loads include berries, apples, and citrus.

We'd like to inspire you to eat eight servings of fruits and vegetables a day to maximize your reproductive health. The average fiber content of fruits and vegetables is about 4 grams per serving. If you eat eight servings a day, you'll be getting about 32 grams of fiber with loads of antioxidants to strengthen sperm and egg quality. That's before you add in legumes and whole grains. Now you can see how easy it will be to exceed 40 grams of fiber per day to optimize the health of your gut microbiome and hormone function and create an anti-inflammatory environment for pregnancy! We advise that you increase your consumption of fiber foods slowly, over a few weeks or months, however. Otherwise, you may experience uncomfortable bloating and gas as your microbiome is stimulated.

Human reproduction is not as efficient as we would like it to be, and in the IVF realm, we often talk about what we can do to optimize embryo quality. Here again, we see that fruits and vegetables are your best bet. A diet with lots of fruits and vegetables provides the bulk of the antioxidants and micronutrients you need to support your health and maximize your fertility. Fruits provide the most antioxidants and vitamin C (of any food group!), while vegetables provide antioxidants, carotenoids, vitamin E, and polyphenols.

Sperm and eggs both accumulate oxidative stress with age,[11,12] and poor diet quality increases free radical production and has the potential to further increase oxidative stress, decrease egg quality, and accelerate egg aging.[13] Fruits and vegetables, which have antioxidant properties, may have the ability to repair or slow down some of the cumulative effects of this oxidative stress on the sperm and eggs. Plant-forward, anti-inflammatory diets can also help reproductive conditions where inflammation plays a larger role such as endometriosis, PCOS, and infertility.

As we saw in chapter one, we have cohort data on what the most fertile women and men eat: a plant-forward diet with lots of fruits, vegetables, whole grains, legumes, seafood, and low amounts of other animal products and processed foods.[14] One novel study compared fruit intake and fast-food intake, and as you can guess, more fruit was associated with a shorter time to pregnancy, while more fast-food meals per week was associated with a longer time to pregnancy.[15] Another study in Brazil looked at more than 2,000 embryos from 269 fertility patients. Not surprising, the embryos from the patients who reported higher intake of vegetables and fruits were of higher quality.[16] These intriguing studies indicate that eating more plants has a positive association with male and female fertility.

Other studies have looked at dietary patterns, miscarriage, and pregnancy complications. One meta-analysis, published in 2023, combined results from six prior studies (two cohort and four case-controls) including a total of more than 13,000 women. Researchers observed a reduction in odds of miscarriage in those who reported a diet abundant in fruits, vegetables, eggs, seafood, dairy, and grains.[17] In another study, women whose diets tended toward a Mediterranean-style eating pattern during pregnancy had lower pregnancy-related adverse outcomes.[18] We'd extend these study findings to say that any plant-forward dietary pattern will most often result in better fertility, reduced miscarriages, and healthier pregnancies.

The Color Chart

Now let's break it down according to the rainbow. Each color of a fruit or vegetable provides different vitamins and minerals.

The Greens

These are the antioxidants you've been looking for! Remember in chapter one how we spoke about oxidative stress, and that antioxidants from foods are your best defense to repair cellular damage? The greens provide the most antioxidants, plus other amazing vitamins and minerals, to benefit your health. Let's discuss a few.

Green vegetables are packed with isoflavones and isothiocyanates, which can enhance immune health and mood, provide energy, and detox the body. All of these tasty green vegetables are low in calories, are nutrient dense, and will help keep your glucose levels stable.

Leafy Greens

You'll get good amounts of folate from each bite of leafy green vegetables. The darker the color, the more nutrients. Dark leafy greens are also the main source of vitamin K1 in our diet. This is a fat-soluble vitamin, which means it is better absorbed when eaten with some fat; adding extra-virgin olive oil to sautéed greens or salad dressing will improve absorption. In addition to its roles assisting with the normal process of blood clotting after an injury and supporting bone metabolism, newer research suggests that vitamin K has antioxidant properties and can rescue some cells from degeneration and cell death.

Calcium is a mineral found in leafy greens. It is important for healthy bones and teeth, and plays a role in cell membrane energy conduction. Calcium is needed for intracellular signaling. It facilitates the acrosome reaction, a necessary step prior to the sperm penetrating the egg. Calcium is also needed for "activation" of the egg, the final step in egg maturation after sperm entry.

Kaempferol is a flavanol found in many plants, with high levels found in kale and spinach. It has strong antioxidant properties to help protect your cells from free radical oxidative damage, which of course is important for eggs and sperm. Kaempferol has been shown to help inhibit cancer cells and reduce the risk of cardiovascular disease by lowering inflammation.

Cruciferous vegetables

Many cruciferous vegetables, members of the brassica family, are also green. These include broccoli, cabbage, kale, and brussels sprouts. They are nutritious powerhouses and provide both men and women with many fertility-promoting nutrients. This family of vegetables is often inexpensive, easily available, nutrient dense, and low in calories. They offer vitamin A, carotenoids, vitamin C, folic acid, and fiber. Besides being anti-inflammatory and great sources of antioxidants, cruciferous vegetables are fabulous for fertility and are great sources of protein, fiber, and even omega-3s. The sulforaphane in cruciferous vegetables has strong anticancer properties as well. Sign us up!

Herbs

We didn't forget about herbs! Herbs are the leaves of some plants that have stronger aromas and flavors. Herbs can have hardy leaves, like rosemary, or delicate leaves, like parsley. They also have antioxidant properties and can really make a dish pop.

Green Fruits and Vegetables

artichoke	celery	kiwi
arugula	cucumber	okra
asparagus	green beans	peas
avocado	green cabbage	romaine lettuce
bok choy	green grapes	spinach
broccoli	green olives	Swiss chard
broccolini	green peppers	zucchini
brussels sprouts	kale	

Herbs

basil	parsley
cilantro	rosemary
dill	sage
mint	tarragon
oregano	thyme

Folate and Pregnancy

Let's take a moment to spotlight folate and its benefits in pregnancy. Folate helps with DNA and RNA synthesis, DNA methylation, cell division, gene expression, protein synthesis, and tissue growth. Folate is the natural form of vitamin B9, and folic acid is the synthetic form. It is found naturally in green leafy vegetables, legumes, grains, and some citrus. Because this vitamin is so critical in early embryo development and some women may not get enough from their diet, additional supplementation with folic acid is recommended pre-pregnancy and during the first trimester to reduce the risk of neural tube defects (NTD) in early fetal development.[19] Eating our fertility diet should provide plenty of folate, especially when combined with folic acid supplementation.

The Reds

Red fruits and vegetables contain powerful antioxidants that are cardioprotective, reduce inflammation, and have anticancer benefits. They are excellent sources of many unique fertility-promoting nutrients.

Colorful beets contain unique betalain phytonutrients that have anti-inflammatory properties and contain many antioxidants. They are an excellent source of vitamin C and manganese (an essential mineral involved in metabolism and bone formation). Betalain pigments in other red plants, such as Swiss chard, rhubarb, amaranth, and cactus fruits, also support your body's natural detoxification processes.

Lycopene is a carotenoid, a plant pigment that adds bright red, yellow, and orange colors to many fruits and vegetables, and is especially beneficial for sperm health. It is an antioxidant that reduces cell damage caused by free radicals and oxidative stress. Adding red fruits and vegetables to your diet can help keep free radical levels in balance. Tomatoes, watermelon, pink grapefruit, papaya, persimmons, and beets, to name a few, are high in lycopene. Cooking tomatoes increases their lycopene content.[20]

Another unique nutrient in red foods is anthocyanin, a different antioxidant found in red, blue, and purple produce. Promising research is finding that this nutrient may help improve oocyte (egg) quality and reduce oxidative stress.

Red Fruits and Vegetables

apples	pomegranates	red peppers
beets	radicchio	rhubarb
cherries	radishes	strawberries
cranberries	raspberries	tomatoes
grapes	red onions	watermelon

The Oranges and Yellows

Oranges and yellows in fruits and vegetables provide carotenoids and flavonoids, including beta-carotene, lutein, and zeaxanthin, which help vision and cell growth. Vitamin C is a water-soluble vitamin that is plentiful in citrus, berries, peppers, and some leafy greens. Vitamin C supports growth, development, and the repair of cells and tissues. It's also a powerful antioxidant that helps reduce cellular damage, supports fertility, and facilitates the absorption of iron. Oranges travel well and are ready to go on their own as a snack. Don't be afraid to toss them in salads or cooked dishes for a naturally sweet flavor accent. One orange a day will meet your body's vitamin C requirement. Citrus contains hesperidin, which helps blood flow and provides nature's best source of vitamin C to boost the immune system.

Yellow fruits and vegetables also provide you with significant sources of fiber, potassium, and vitamin B6. Sweet potatoes fall into this category. There are a number of varieties available, and they have a lower glycemic index and more nutrients than white or yellow potatoes.

Beta-carotene is the precursor to vitamin A and is found in orange fruits and vegetables such as carrots and melons. These compounds are most known to support vision. They are also important for growth and cell division, key to the health of an early embryo and fetus. Vitamin A has antioxidant properties and can protect cells against free radical damage. One serving of winter squash, sweet potatoes, or pumpkin will meet your vitamin A requirements for two days! These delicious and easy-to-prepare vegetables taste sweet and savory. As a bonus, their fiber helps to balance blood sugar.

Orange and Yellow Fruits and Vegetables

bananas	mangoes	summer squash
cantaloupe	orange peppers	sweet potatoes
carrots	oranges	winter squash (acorn,
corn	papayas	butternut, delicata,
ginger	peaches	kabocha)
grapefruit	pineapple	yellow peppers
golden beets	pumpkin	
lemon	salmonberries	

The Purples and Blues

Bright purples and blues contain anthocyanins and resveratrol, antioxidants that can reduce oxidative stress and repair cell damage. They also provide vitamin K, manganese, and vitamin C. The antioxidant powers of purple and blue fruits and vegetables can help with producing healthy egg and sperm, reduce inflammation to promote a healthy uterine lining, and improve insulin sensitivity.[21]

Anthocyanins deserve a special shout-out. A subtype of dietary flavonoids that have significant antioxidant properties,[22] they are found in certain vegetables and fruits, tea, chocolate, and wine. Quite a few of the purple and blue fruit and vegetable group, including mulberries, black raspberries, pomegranates, red onions, red cabbage, eggplant, and purple sweet potatoes, contain anthocyanins. Anthocyanins demonstrate anticancer and antiaging properties, have cardioprotective benefits, and may help prevent cognitive decline. Anthocyanins in these fruits and vegetables help to manage blood pressure, cholesterol levels, and glucose levels along with reducing inflammation in your body. For example, eating blueberries contributes to a reduction in oxidative stress, which has been shown to prevent cardiovascular disease, benefit diabetes management, suppress visceral fat accumulation, manage elevated cholesterol levels, and protect against many gastric, urinary tract, eye, and nervous system diseases. Whew! These foods pack quite a punch!

Purple and Blue Fruits and Vegetables

blackberries	purple kale	purple cauliflowers
blueberries	plums	purple peppers
cherries	prunes	purple potatoes
eggplant	purple cabbage	red or purple grapes
figs	purple carrots	

Try Something New!

Never had a pomegranate? How about a persimmon? What about broccolini? Leeks? Fennel? Shallots? Purple cauliflower? Asian pear? Beets? Now is your time to experiment. Each time you shop, buy at least seven to ten fruits and vegetables that you are familiar with, plus one new fruit or vegetable. Head home and make a plan to eat it. Check out some of the recipes from this book or search online. Include your partner, friends, or family in your cooking-new-foods adventure. It will be fun! Plan a Saturday or Sunday event to try something new. Be adventurous in your eating!

The Whites

The white fruit and vegetable group, which includes alliums like garlic and onions, and some cruciferous vegetables like cauliflower, contains organosulfur compounds and quercetin, which are great boosters for the immune system, providing antiviral, antibacterial, and anticancer properties. Onions, garlic, and shallots include polyphenols along with vitamin C. Garlic and onions also include sulfur-containing amino acids and peptides that support our cellular detoxification systems.

Alliums contain antioxidants including vitamin C, vitamin B, folate, selenium, potassium, and manganese, as well as anti-inflammatory properties to support fertility. Soluble fiber in alliums contains fructans, which promote the health of the gut microbiome. The flavonoids in alliums produce glutathione, which is a very powerful antioxidant to remove toxins. Quercetin is a flavonoid great at reducing inflammation.

White Vegetables

cauliflower	jicama	potatoes
daikon radish	leeks	scallions
fennel	onions	shallots
garlic	parsnips	turnips

What About Mushrooms?

Although they grow in the ground, mushrooms are not a plant. Technically speaking, mushrooms are fungi. There are thousands of varieties of mushrooms. The most common edible ones include cremini, portobello, shiitake, chantarelle, porcini, lobster, button or white, enoki, maitake, and oyster. Mushrooms contain many helpful micronutrients such as selenium, magnesium, copper, zinc, potassium, and B vitamins. Mushrooms left in the sun and exposed to ultraviolet light can produce vitamin D.

Mushrooms have long been revered for their health benefits, which are quite extensive. They can slow cell damage and support cardiovascular, brain, and immune health. They lower blood pressure, protect nerves, and support blood glucose, gastrointestinal and liver health, and mood. They are being studied for their anticancer properties as well.

The general antioxidant and anti-inflammatory properties of mushrooms support many aspects of reproductive health. The beta-glucan soluble dietary fiber can lower cholesterol, decrease inflammation, and help to regulate blood sugar, reducing insulin resistance. B vitamins help produce energy and support metabolic reactions. Pantothenic acid, or vitamin B5, helps with synthesis of coenzyme A, a cofactor for many metabolic processes, and with the formation of hormones. Potassium helps with blood pressure, which is important when the placenta is starting to develop and throughout pregnancy. Selenium prevents cell damage and is important for thyroid health and sperm motility; it plays an important role in reproductive health and growth and development of the fetus in pregnancy. Zinc supports DNA synthesis, gene expression, growth and development, and sperm health.

Shopping for Fruits and Vegetables

When you can, eat locally sourced vegetables in season for the highest nutrient density. Although it is possible to buy almost any vegetable year-round due to international farming and shipping, fruits and vegetables bought in season and from closer farms will taste better and be more nutritious. For example, asparagus is at its best in the spring in North America, not the fall when it is shipped from another hemisphere. Quite a bit of the nutritional value can be lost when vegetables are harvested early and shipped halfway across the globe. Hardy leafy greens and root vegetables grow year-round in many climates, but colder months can be a challenge in some areas, with less variety available. This is when frozen produce can come in handy. Frozen produce is harvested at its peak and frozen before shipping so not much is lost as far as nutrients or taste is concerned.

If you have the option, shopping at your local farmers market in the spring, summer, and fall is a pure delight. You'll have an opportunity to talk with farmers and discover more about seed varieties, heirloom crops, and the season's harvest. We especially love going to the farmers market in the height of summer and seeing all the different types of lettuces that are so bright and voluminous. Take a chance and try whatever looks the most bountiful that week! Bite a raw leaf, without any topping. How does the flavor compare to others you have had? When you buy leafy greens, look for firm, unbruised leaves and stems. Some of the lettuce greens are more delicate.

Many people enjoy tending their own vegetable and herb gardens, as they gain the advantage of eating the ripest produce, bursting with flavor and nutrients. If you like to garden, greens are very easy to grow, even in the colder months. Common greens include multiple varieties of kale such as green, purple, Lacinato (or dino) kale; Swiss or rainbow chard; spinach; green, purple, or Napa cabbage; collard greens; and beet greens. It is easy to keep the hardier greens in your freezer, such as a bag of frozen spinach or kale, to throw into a soup or smoothie. Excess kale from your garden can be blanched and frozen. Leafy greens are also inexpensive relative to most vegetables. They can last up to one to two weeks in the refrigerator.

Is there a difference between boxed or bagged greens and a full head of lettuce? Nutritionally, there probably isn't a big one, although prepackaged versions are likely prepped in a way to extend their shelf life compared to fresh. Once the box or bag is opened, the leaves will age more quickly. If you are shopping sustainably, it's ideal to skip the extra plastic packaging, but the convenience of products like prepackaged, boxed lettuce is hard to beat. Make sure to look at the sell-by date and see that the leaves look fresh. You may notice that a full head of organic lettuce has more flavor than the boxed varieties. On the other hand, the boxed and bagged greens require less time to prep, so you may be more likely to eat them daily. We usually keep both on hand.

Organic Versus Conventionally Grown Produce

When you are trying to conceive, it's ideal to limit exposures to toxins, including herbicides and pesticides. Some of these substances can persist in our bodies and reduce fertility.[23] So should everyone always buy organic if it's available? Not necessarily. Organic produce usually costs more, and we never want to see someone eat fewer fruits and vegetables because the organic variety is too expensive. We would always rather see you buy a large assortment of traditionally grown fruits and vegetables and rinse them well before eating. Plus, even organic fruits and vegetables contain trace amounts of pesticides.

No matter what kind of produce you buy, rinsing before eating will reduce your chance of getting a foodborne illness and dilute any residual pesticides. Organic produce and even prewashed boxed or bagged lettuce could harbor bacteria from contaminated water sources and should be rinsed. The positive correlation with eating more fruits and vegetables and higher fertility means you should focus on eating lots of fruits and veggies every day and worry less about whether or not they are organic. So pick out a variety of veggies, rinse, and enjoy! The benefits far outweigh the risks.

Preparing and Cooking Vegetables

We want you to think about how you cook and consume vegetables so you can include more of them in your meals. You can eat them raw, steam them, blend them in a smoothie, sauté them, or toss them into a stew.

Eaten raw, all enzymes and water-soluble vitamins are preserved. Try them this way alone or with a hummus dip for maximum nutrient value. Cooking vegetables can reduce some of their health benefits, but again, it's better to eat vegetables that are cooked and seasoned to your liking rather than not eat them at all. Consider including a mix of cooked and raw vegetables in a dish by finishing it with some raw radishes, arugula, or herbs.

Should you peel your vegetables? Not necessarily. The skin, or peel, of the vegetable has more fiber and is dense in vitamins. The skin of some root vegetables like carrots, sweet potatoes, and turnips, may have a more bitter flavor profile. Taste to find out! Whether or not you peel, you should still plan to wash the skins under cool water before preparing.

Culinary Spotlight: *Mise en Place*

Mise en place is a good term to get familiar with and practice. It is a French culinary term meaning "everything in its place." The idea is that you have prepped and assembled all the ingredients for your meal and have laid them out in order before you start cooking. That way, the cooking can progress in an organized fashion, allowing each step the correct amount of cooking time without interruption. Once this becomes a habit, the cooking itself is quick and easy. It is truly a secret of professional chefs and great home cooks alike!

For more complex dishes, you can often start by dicing and sautéing a classic grouping of vegetables to create a flavor profile, then add cooked beans or lentils to make a meal. Here are a few of our favorites:

From France, *mirepoix*: onions, carrots, celery
From Spain, *sofrito*: onions, bell pepper, tomato
From India: ginger, garlic, green chilis
From Mexico: onions, tomato, garlic
From Louisiana, United States: onions, green bell pepper, celery

When it comes to the actual cooking, the degree of heat applied to vegetables will affect their nutrient content. Steaming may enhance some nutrients such as lycopene in tomatoes and beta-carotene in carrots. As heat increases, some nutrients will be lost. For example, steaming broccoli for up to five minutes retains the most benefit, versus boiling, which allows more nutrients to leach out.[24] Vegetables can be quickly blanched, which may brighten their color and be more appealing for a crudité plate or midday snacking. Dry heat cooking may include grilling, roasting, sautéing, or stir-frying. Grilling may lose only a small amount of nutrients. Sautéing or stir-frying vegetables may result in small nutrient loss but preserve most. Roasting may result in more vitamins being lost while preserving minerals. In general, you don't have to worry too much about losing nutrients if you eat a variety of vegetables prepared in different ways throughout the course of a week.

Fertility Greens

Cooking greens is ridiculously simple. If you've got any of the hardier greens, you can make what we call Fertility Greens! These are so easy, it barely counts as a recipe. It's ten minutes to get your daily greens in. Simply remove the leaves from the ribs, tear them into smaller pieces, and rinse them. You can even leave the stems on if you like the crunch. Then, put them in a pot or skillet with a small amount of water and steam for three to five minutes until wilted, stirring occasionally directly in the pan. Pull them out and put them on a beautiful plate. Drizzle with some high-quality extra-virgin olive oil, squeeze on some fresh lemon juice, and sprinkle with finishing salt. Delicious!

Cooking Mushrooms

The umami flavor of mushrooms creates a sense of satisfaction and satiety and can function as a meat replacement. The many varieties of mushrooms have quite a range of flavors, well beyond the traditional white button mushrooms. Sautéing porcini, chanterelle, or lobster mushrooms in some olive oil with a dash of salt is a delicious side dish or salad topping. Making a risotto with chanterelles, sage, and winter squash is a much more nutritious comfort food than traditional macaroni and cheese. Grilling or roasting a portobello, basting it with olive oil and balsamic vinegar and placing it atop a bed of greens, or smothering it with roasted poblanos, a slice of tomato, and some feta, can serve as a delicious burger alternative. Some types of mushrooms are quite expensive, so we count some of these unique types as a delicacy. When the fall comes and mushrooms have been locally foraged, be sure to try a few specialty ones from your local farmers market or grocery.

Culinary Spotlight: Salt and MSG

Salt is an essential component in cooking and flavoring foods. It can bring a dish together to create harmony. For the recipes in our book, we use Diamond Crystal kosher salt unless otherwise specified, but any salt will do. Just make sure you know how "salty" your salt tastes, so you can begin to intuit how much to add as you cook. Typically, salt is added at each step in the cooking process. It is especially important to help bring out the flavor of vegetables. If salt is left out during cooking, the finished dish may taste flat or bland. If salt is appropriately added during cooking, less finishing salt is needed, and the dish will have less sodium overall.

Individuals perceive tastes differently, including their preference for saltiness or heat. For this reason, we are not offended if someone wants to add a little salt or hot sauce at the table to enhance their enjoyment of a dish. For a finishing salt, we prefer Maldon sea salt or Himalayan pink salt. Keep in mind, these salts with bigger flakes bring out both the savory and sweet flavors of a dish, but do not contain iodine like the more typical iodized table salt.

Another flavor enhancer is monosodium glutamate (MSG), the sodium salt of the amino acid glutamate. Glutamate occurs naturally in foods such as mushrooms, Parmesan cheese, fish, meat, seaweed, and tomatoes. MSG was first isolated from seaweed in Japan in the early 1900s. Historically, it's gotten a bad rap as people blamed it for symptoms they had after eating in Chinese restaurants, but this association is now recognized as a myth. Negative reactions to MSG are rare, and it is in fact now lauded for its benefit in the culinary world. MSG can increase the essence of taste, or umami, in foods. Using a little MSG can have an almost magical effect, enhancing the vegetable flavor of vegetables and allowing you to reduce your added salt. This can be especially beneficial for individuals trying to reduce their sodium intake but who don't want their food to taste bland. It can make a carrot taste more carroty! Try it in some vegetable dishes that don't have much natural glutamate and see if you notice a difference.

Nutritional Spotlight: Iodine

Iodine is needed to make thyroid hormone. Lack of iodine can lead to a condition called hypothyroidism, or an underperforming thyroid. Symptoms of thyroid deficiency include feeling weak or tired, weight gain, constipation, dry skin, and hair loss. It has also been linked to irregular ovulation and miscarriage. (Note that you can also develop subclinical hypothyroidism, which is when your thyroid gland is beginning to underperform but clinical symptoms of deficiency are not present.) Adequate intake of 150 milligrams (mg) of iodine daily preconception is recommended to support thyroid function, and 220 milligrams daily is recommended during pregnancy. Make sure you have an adequate intake of iodine to avoid deficiency. Iodine may be obtained from foods such as fish, seaweed, or dairy, iodized salt, or a prenatal vitamin.

Getting More Fruits and Vegetables into Your Diet

How can anyone eat eight servings of fruits and vegetables a day? If this sounds like a much larger amount than what you may be currently eating, don't worry—we'll tell you how you can easily increase your numbers. Think about adding them to every meal and snack, including breakfast. Remember, vegetables should take up half your "plate." Throw greens into a breakfast scramble. Eat some cucumber or tomatoes on the side of a bowl of oatmeal. Add spinach or kale into a breakfast smoothie. For snacks, prepare sliced veggies such as peppers, cucumbers, carrots, celery, or snap peas and have them easily available. Add some hummus or white bean dip for some protein and even more fiber.

Leave fresh fruits on your counter to snack on anytime. At lunch, enjoy a big salad featuring vegetables and fruits of many colors. Consider vegetable-based soups or bowls. You can easily prepare a bowl with lettuce, whole grains, and other vegetables or beans. Use leftover veggies from dinner the night before for lunch or snacks. After work, have a veggie appetizer or a cup of soup while you are preparing dinner. For dinner, plan to prepare at least three vegetables to fill half your plate and have leftovers for tomorrow's lunch. Eating a salad every day, for lunch or dinner, is an easy way to get a variety of vegetables and leafy greens into your diet. When you plan ahead, it becomes easy to get more servings of vegetables daily.

There are many other resources out there to help in your goal of increasing your fruit and vegetable intake. The U.S. Army Office of the Surgeon General uses the best available sports science to offer advice on healthy nutrition, including eight servings of fruits and vegetables a day. Their website has some great ideas you can use to increase your fruits and vegetables such as adding vegetables to omelets, using spaghetti squash instead of pasta noodles, or making mashed cauliflower.[25] The Mayo Clinic has a 1-2-3 plan to help you get at least six servings of fruits and vegetables a day: one at breakfast, two at lunch, and three at dinner.[26] Add in a couple more as snacks, and you are up to your eight!

Tips for the Grocery

Most of us shop at grocery stores every week. One thing to keep in mind: the freshest foods are stocked at the perimeter, where they are easily accessible for frequent deliveries. That's where you want to do most of your shopping, too. Fruits, vegetables, dairy, eggs, tofu, fish, and meat are all located there. The exception is of course beans and lentils, which you'll find in the bulk section or stocked on shelves.

Shop with a list and be aware of the signals that grocers and the food industry use to get our attention. Foods that are at eye level, foods at the ends of the aisles, and candy at the checkout are all designed to get us to put extra items in our cart. And try to avoid shopping when hungry, since this is when we are more likely to be persuaded by those easy-to-grab, hyperpalatable snacks.

Salad Anytime: The Five Components of a Simple, Delicious Salad

Throwing a salad together with ingredients on hand is so easy if you can remember this simple combination: something green, something crunchy, something sweet, something savory, and something sour.

Start with whatever greens you have on hand. Add nuts or a crunchy vegetable such as cucumber, radish, and kohlrabi. Add fresh fruit like strawberries or pomegranate seeds, or dried fruit like cranberries. To finish, top with your home-made dressing (keep reading for a super simple and flavorful dressing recipe). Keep some fresh herbs around such as parsley, cilantro, and mint to add some zest to your salad. For an optional umami component: sprinkle on a small amount of cheese such as feta, goat cheese, or blue cheese.

Making your own dressing is super easy and so much better for you. Take a good extra-virgin olive oil (EVOO) and add vinegar or lemon juice. Vinegars each have unique flavor profiles—try starting with red wine, balsamic, or apple cider. Mix in a 3:1 or 2:1 EVOO to vinegar ratio, depending on your preference. Add sea salt and freshly ground pepper. Fresh dressing, no additives! You can mix in some Dijon mustard, which is great with spinach salad, or fresh lemon juice for a Caesar salad.

For an additional texture element, consider adding sprouts. Seeds that have germinated and sprouted, sprouts are full of vitamins, minerals, and anti-oxidants. Add a handful to a salad or grain bowl for a green, earthy texture. You can easily grow them yourself at home or buy sprouts at a grocery or farmers market. Start with alfalfa or broccoli sprouts, and, from there, you can try other seeds or legumes for different flavors.

Massaged Kale Salad with Citrus and Pomegranate (V, GF)

Prep time: 20 minutes

Total time: 20 minutes

Yield: *4 to 6 servings*

1 bunch Lacinato kale, stems removed, torn into large pieces

1 teaspoon sea salt (iodized)

¼ cup extra-virgin olive oil

2 tablespoons apple cider vinegar

1 blood orange or small navel orange, peeled and sliced into thin rounds

½ cup pomegranate seeds

¼ cup toasted walnuts or other nuts

Ground pepper (optional), to taste

2 ounces goat cheese or feta cheese (optional)

Substitutions for pomegranate seeds: strawberries, dried cranberries, or cherries

This massaged kale salad was a class favorite. Ripping the leaves from the stems, tearing the leaves into bite-sized pieces, and massaging them with a little salt gives you permission to enjoy touching the greens as you prepare them, much in the way you might let warm sand run through your hands as you lounge on a beach in the summer. Plus, massaging the kale decreases the bitterness and softens it, too. Delicious all year, this kale salad can be adapted to the season. During the winter, it pairs well with citrus. The vitamin C from citrus increases our ability to absorb iron from the kale. Pomegranates are high in vitamin C and polyphenols, power antioxidants. In the summer, substitute ripe strawberries. If you don't have fresh fruit available, substitute dried cranberries. Olive oil helps the body absorb the fat-soluble vitamins in this luscious salad, and the nuts add omega-3 fatty acids, zinc, and magnesium, which benefit fertility for women and men.

1. Place kale in a large bowl and sprinkle sea salt on top. Using your hands, massage the kale leaves, working the salt into the leaves. If you've got some large leaves, tear them into smaller pieces as you go. Continue to massage for about 5 minutes,

until kale has turned a vibrant green and softened. Set aside for at least 10 minutes.

2. In a small bowl, whisk together the olive oil and apple cider vinegar. Pour over the kale and toss to coat.

3. Top the kale with blood oranges, pomegranate seeds, walnuts, and a little bit of black pepper. If desired, sprinkle with goat cheese or feta.

Now you're ready for a more complex recipe! You can put your newfound knowledge of vegetables and culinary skills into a delicious one-pan meal.

Quinoa Vegetable Paella (V, VG, DF, GF)

Prep time: 15 minutes
Cook time: 30 minutes
Total time: 45 minutes

Yield: 6 servings

½ teaspoon saffron threads
1 tablespoon warm water
1 tablespoon extra-virgin
    olive oil
1 medium onion, peeled and
    chopped
1 red bell pepper, seeded and
    diced
3 garlic cloves, peeled and
    minced
1 cup quinoa, rinsed
1 (15-ounce) can or box
    chickpeas, drained and
    rinsed
1 (14.5-ounce) can or box
    diced tomatoes, fire
    roasted
1 (14-ounce) jar artichoke
    hearts, quartered
1 teaspoon smoked paprika
2 cups vegetable broth
Salt and pepper
1 cup fresh or frozen peas

The national dish of Spain, paella is a lovely, flavorful rice dish. Variations of paella highlight the bounty of the Mediterranean, classically featuring shellfish and meat. This nutrient-dense, all-plant version uses quinoa instead of rice and chickpeas for protein and highlights different vegetables for their unique colors and nutrients: red tomatoes with lycopene; white onions with vitamin C, B6, and folate; and green peas for vitamin K and protein. Saffron is a powerful antioxidant. The paprika and red pepper both contain capsaicin, which has antioxidant properties and improves immunity. Each bite bursts with flavor and texture! You won't believe how easy it is to prepare as a one-skillet dish. Note: Saffron is a specialty spice and can be rather pricey. It is a classic part of paella and can add a deeper complexity to the dish, but if you do not have it on hand, feel free to leave it out.

1. Combine saffron threads and 1 tablespoon warm water in a small bowl. Set aside for 10 minutes.
2. Heat the oil in a large skillet over medium heat. Add the onion and red pepper and a pinch of salt, sautéing until onions are translucent, about 2 minutes. Add garlic and cook 2 more minutes.
3. Add quinoa, chickpeas, tomatoes (with their liquid), artichoke hearts, paprika,

and the saffron mixture into the skillet. Add the vegetable broth and a pinch of salt and pepper, and stir again to incorporate.

4. Bring the mixture to a boil, then cover and reduce to a simmer for 20 to 25 minutes, until most of the liquid has been absorbed.

5. Remove the lid and stir in the peas. Cover again and simmer for another 10 minutes. Salt to taste.

Kitchen Tip: You can prepare 2 cups of chickpeas from scratch in place of canned or boxed.

Revati's Story

Revati started trying to conceive the year after she got married. Growing up in India, she described herself as always being a bit "pudgy." Her mother worked, and maybe out of guilt, or not knowing what good nutrition was, she would frequently indulge Revati with chocolates and cake. Her typical Indian meals consisted of breads and rice, with dal, and vegetable and meat curries.

When Revati went in for an evaluation, she was diagnosed with PCOS. Her husband also received a diagnosis of male factor infertility. They tried IVF first in India, but it failed. She decided to move to the United States because the medical care was better, and she knew in her heart how much she wanted a family. She had been to astrologists in India who told her she would not have a baby and she should just focus on her career, which brought her to tears. She was determined to fight their readings.

Once they settled in Seattle, Revati saw a reproductive endocrinologist who recommended our Food for Fertility class before attempting more IVF cycles. During the class, she learned how to approach new vegetables and salads. She was especially enamored with kale, chard, and broccoli. She learned how to make a full meal of a salad with a combination of greens, grains, nuts, veggies, and fruits. She stopped eating bread in the morning. The class motivated her to walk more and to use resistance bands for some strength exercise. She lost ten pounds by making simple, nonrestrictive changes.

She was determined to get pregnant and tried IVF two more times. She had two miscarriages and briefly considered surrogacy or donor eggs, but she found herself unwilling to give up. She saw a high-risk OB specialist who recommended some additional medications to reduce her risk of miscarriage. With her next frozen embryo transfer, she had a positive pregnancy test, used the additional medications, and went on to successfully deliver her son.

She had developed gestational diabetes during the pregnancy, which was controlled with diet and oral medication. She continued to eat well after pregnancy and joined a gym to commit to treating her diabetes with a healthy lifestyle. Her husband joined her in working out and eating more healthfully, and he also lost weight.

She began having regular periods, whereas before they had always been irregular from the PCOS. Later that year, her period was five days late. She couldn't believe it; she was almost forty. After fourteen years of struggling with infertility, how could she possibly have a spontaneous pregnancy? But it was true. She had done it on her own. Thanks largely to her diet and lifestyle changes, her PCOS symptoms had improved. This time she was pregnant with a girl, born nineteen months after her son.

She glows when she tells me how her son eats "all the vegetables," loves broccoli, and doesn't eat any sweets. She is planning to feed her daughter similarly, to hopefully minimize her risk for PCOS. Revati credits her success to her motivation, determination, and her personal team, the people who supported her through her long journey: her mother, friends, her support group, her fertility doctor and high-risk OB specialist, her fertility nurse, her dietitian, her acupuncturist, and most importantly, her husband. Her advice: "Don't give up on your dream."

Takeaways

1. Different colors of fruits and vegetables indicate different phyto-nutrients. By eating a variety, you maximize the antioxidants and anti-inflammatory effects.
2. A plant-forward diet has been shown to improve the quality of sperm, eggs, and embryos. Women and men who eat a plant-forward, whole-food diet with more fruits and vegetables have better outcomes with IVF.
3. For best fertility, mood, and gut health, aim for seven to eight servings of fruits and vegetables per day.

Sample SMART Goals

1. Try your hand at a salad using these five components: something green, something crunchy, something sweet, something savory, and something sour.
2. Eat something with cooked tomatoes.
3. Try a new fruit or vegetable each week.
4. Make fruits easily available by keeping them on the counter.
5. Blanch and prep some broccoli and carrots for snacks throughout the week.
6. Gamify it! Aim to eat eight different fruits and vegetables daily.
7. Eat fresh berries when they are in season and frozen berries when they are not.

Chapter 4

Whole Grains: Fuel Foods

Test Your Knowledge

Gluten is inflammatory and bad for fertility.* True/False

Low-carbohydrate diets are healthy for fertility.** True/False

G rains have become one of our society's most controversial foods, with some even suggesting that they should be avoided. But *whole* grains, in contrast to processed grains like all-purpose white flour, provide essential nutrients and fiber that are key to your diet when you are trying to conceive. We'll explain the difference in how grains are processed, the difference between simple and complex carbohydrates, and what causes a high versus low glucose response. After this chapter, you will be a much

---

* False. Gluten is a *protein* found in wheat, barley, and rye grains. If you have celiac disease, an autoimmune disease, or are sensitive to gluten, you need to avoid gluten. If you don't have these health problems but avoid gluten anyway, you may be missing out on fertility-promoting vitamins, fiber, and minerals. Some people think that since gluten is inflammatory for celiac disease it is inflammatory for everyone. If you have celiac disease, strictly avoid gluten and be sure to include high-fiber, gluten-free grains such as quinoa or buckwheat in your diet.

** False. Your body's preferred source of energy are carbohydrates. Research and our patients' experience have shown that a plant-forward, high-fiber diet improves fertility.

better consumer of grains and you won't have to worry about going "low carb."

Health Benefits

Whole grains are high in fiber, vitamin E, selenium, and lignans, which are precursors to phytoestrogens. Eating a diet containing whole grains is beneficial for everyone, as they decrease inflammation and the risk for chronic diseases. Whole grains have been shown to reduce the risk of cardiovascular disease, colon cancer, and all-cause mortality. In one of the largest studies of cardiovascular risk factors, the Framingham Offspring Cohort Study published in 2004, individuals who ate higher whole grains and fiber had lower insulin resistance, reducing their risk of diabetes.[1] In addition, intake of whole grains lowers systemic inflammation and defends against reactive oxygen species.

Fertility Benefits

Whole grains hit all three of the factors that make them strong supporters of fertility. They are anti-inflammatory, they are low glycemic, and they contain many antioxidants. Their high fiber content feeds the gut microbiome, which, as we know, supports fertility. Studies have demonstrated that people who incorporate whole grains into their diet are more fertile and live longer.

Specific micronutrients found in whole grains that are good for reproductive health include B vitamins, magnesium, copper, zinc, and iron. Men who eat whole grains that are low glycemic have better sperm quality and higher fertility on average.[2] The anti-inflammatory and insulin-sensitizing benefits are especially good for women with PCOS or recurrent pregnancy loss. Antioxidants in whole grains also promote fertility by reducing oxidative stress in sperm and eggs. Too much oxidation can potentially alter mitochondrial function or cause DNA damage within eggs and sperm.

In a study of food intake in patients undergoing IVF, those with the highest intake of whole grains had a higher rate of implantation and live birth.[3] Each additional serving of whole grains intake was correlated with a 0.4 millimeter thicker endometrial lining, leading to better endometrial receptivity.

Celiac Disease and Gluten Sensitivity

Gluten is the main protein in wheat and is what gives bread its elastic texture. About 4 percent of the population may be sensitive or intolerant to gluten, and about 1 to 2 percent have celiac disease. Celiac disease causes damage to the villi in the small intestine, which can reduce the absorption of key nutrients for fertility such as folic acid, iron, and vitamin D. Although rare, undiagnosed celiac disease can be a cause of infertility.

Individuals with celiac disease and those with gluten sensitivity should avoid wheat, barley, rye, and other gluten-containing grains to prevent an inflammatory response. Seek out gluten-free grains. These include many of the ancient grains—varieties of whole grains that have been around for thousands of years that are high in fiber and micronutrients, and provide an excellent source of energy—such as quinoa, buckwheat (which is not wheat, despite the name), sorghum, amaranth, and millet. Many processed gluten-free bread products can be low in fiber and nutritional quality, so try to be mindful of that. Thankfully, there are many whole grains that are nutrient dense that do not contain gluten at all.

Whole Grains with Gluten

barley	freekeh	spelt
bulgur	kamut	wheat berries
emmer farro	rye berries	

Whole Grains Without Gluten

amaranth	corn	red rice
black rice	millet	sorghum
brown rice	oats	teff
buckwheat	quinoa	white rice

Everyday Wheat Versus Whole Grains

Why does it seem that so many people are having a problem with wheat in the United States? Is there truly a rise in gluten intolerance and inflammation due to wheat? Could the issue be the genetics of the modern wheat strain, or the herbicide Roundup (glyphosate) that is applied to most commercial wheat crops to increase the yield? Or is it what is missing from most conventional wheat—the fiber?

The type of grains available to most U.S. consumers has changed since the Green Revolution in the mid-twentieth century. Initially envisioned to alleviate world hunger, strains of wheat were chosen for maximum yield. These choices have resulted in some unfortunate downsides as well. The shift to monoculture farming requires the use of more fertilizers and pesticides, resulting in soil depletion and loss of ecological biodiversity.

The milling has changed, too. Industrial wheat in the United States is steel milled, allowing the fiber-containing bran to be more easily removed, creating the fine, shelf-stable white flour with which we are all familiar. Commercial all-purpose flour, and most processed bread, pasta, and snack foods, contain this depleted wheat.

We encourage you to look past everyday wheat and discover the ancient grains. Ancient grains can be eaten whole, or stone-milled the old-fashioned way, preserving the bran and germ to feed your gut microbiome the fiber it needs.

Whole Grains Versus Processed/Refined/ Enriched Grains

Whole grains are composed of three parts: the bran, the endosperm, and the germ. The bran, or outer shell, contains fiber, B vitamins, magnesium, copper, zinc, iron, and antioxidants. The endosperm contains carbohydrates, some protein, and some vitamins and minerals. The inner germ contains protein, vitamin E, minerals, and B vitamins. Whole grains, with all three parts, provide sustainable energy and nutrients for an active lifestyle.

We get "refined grains" when the bran and the germ are removed from whole grains, leaving only the starchy endosperm. These refined grains are used to make flour but have fewer nutrients. Many grocery products such as bread, pasta, cereals, and crackers contain less-nutritious, stripped-down, refined grains. Refined grains become "enriched" grains, sometimes called "fortified" grains, if folic acid and other B vitamins are added back in. However, neither enriched nor fortified grains are as nutritious as the whole grain they started from.

Ultra-Processed Foods

Walk into any grocery store and you will be bombarded with multiple rows of ultra-processed foods. These foods now make up an average of 60 percent of the daily energy intake for most U.S. consumers.[4] Ultra-processed foods can harm your fertility because they typically contain refined grains that increase inflammation (due to their lack of fiber) and crowd out the nutrients your body needs from whole foods for cells to function optimally. Many heavily processed foods also have a high glycemic index, which can spike your blood sugar and increase insulin resistance—think potato chips, French fries, tortilla chips, pretzels, cookies, cakes, baked goods, energy drinks, coffee drinks, and sodas. The effect of these foods on your health is likely related to how frequently you consume them and how much space they are taking up in your diet, squeezing out fiber- and nutrient-rich vegetables and legumes. When eating ultra-processed foods or processed grains, remember intuitive eating principles. These foods aren't off limits, but slow down and savor each bite. An occasional snack food or beverage is probably not much of a problem, but when these foods make up a significant proportion of your energy intake, they are likely causing harm. And, as proven by many studies, eating ultra-processed foods can inadvertently result in higher calorie consumption and weight gain due to their hyper-palatability.[5] We recommend keeping ultra-processed foods to less than 10 percent of your daily intake.

Unfriend the Snack Food and Fast-Food Industries

How can you reduce processed foods when they are so ubiquitous? First and foremost, become a savvy consumer. Be aware of advertising and sizing, and realize that more is not always better. Limit eating out. We know that when people cook at home, meals are more nutrient dense and lower in calories. Compared to eating out at fast casual restaurants, eating at home can also save you money.

When choosing to eat out occasionally, set yourself up for success by starting your meal with vegetables or a salad. The fiber will start to fill you up. Portion sizes are usually larger in restaurants than what you serve yourself at home, so consider ordering an appetizer as your main dish. Or cut a full-size portion in half, and plan to take leftovers home for lunch the next day. Of course, if you are eating intuitively and are still hungry, by all means, eat more! This is not about restriction or reduction, but a recognition of larger portion sizes in some restaurants. Many of us eat what is put in front of us and don't tune into our hunger and satiety signals. We want you to be a competent eater and recognize your internal cues!

You can also use behavioral science to your advantage by creating obstacles or distractions for foods you want to eat less often. This means not keeping chips and soda in the house, avoiding passing by vending machines, and not driving down the street with the fast-food restaurants on your way home.

Simple Carbs / Complex Carbs and Glycemic Index / Glycemic Load

Any grains that have been refined, including enriched or fortified grains, are known as simple carbohydrates. The process of removing the bran and germ removes the fiber part of the grain and transforms it from a nutritionally rich complex carb to a rather pedestrian simple carb. For many people, the digestive process is accelerated for simple carbs, causing a faster rise in blood sugar, and a faster fall after insulin secretion. We often have too many of these refined grains in our diet.

Whole grains, or complex carbohydrates, by contrast, are not a problem for your body. This is largely thanks to the natural presence of fiber, which slows down the absorption of glucose and keeps blood sugar levels more even. Because whole grains retain their fiber, they have a lower glycemic index than refined grains. The glycemic index refers to how high your blood sugar rises after you eat a certain food. The glycemic load is a similar tool used to assess glucose response to foods, taking into account how much total carbohydrate is in a given serving. Some fruits, like watermelon, for instance, may have a high glycemic index but a low glycemic load, meaning the overall amount of sugar in a typical serving size is relatively small, since it contains mainly water.

The glucose response after ingestion of carbohydrates can vary quite a bit between individuals, likely due to differences in their genetic expression and microbiomes. For most people, carbohydrates with a lower glycemic load and more fiber (whole foods) will result in a lower spike in blood sugar. If you are consuming mainly whole foods made up of complex carbohydrates, you don't need to worry about the glycemic index or the glycemic load of foods. Gluten presence or absence does not affect the glycemic response. What matters is whether the grain has undergone processing that removes the fiber. By sticking to whole grains and whole fruits and vegetables, you will not need to worry about blood sugar spikes and resulting inflammation.

Whole grains = complex carbohydrates with high fiber
Low to medium glycemic index

Refined, fortified, or enriched grains = simple carbohydrates with low fiber
Medium to high glycemic index

Women with PCOS, prediabetes, and type 2 diabetes sometimes hear the message that they should avoid all carbohydrates to avoid raising blood sugar. If the recommendations were more specific, they would understand this applies only to refined simple carbohydrates, not whole grains. Any foods where the fiber has been removed, including most grocery store breads and pasta, are considered high glycemic. Consumption of these simple carbohydrates should be limited and, when eaten, paired with something high in fiber (nut butter or bean dip) to curb the blood sugar spike. Although this recommendation holds for everyone, people with diabetes need to pay closer attention to reducing simple carbs and high glycemic foods.

For many individuals, white rice is a dietary staple. It is a simple carb, which has had the bran and germ removed. Typically, white rice is eaten with other foods such as vegetables, beans, lentils, or small portions of meat that decrease the glucose spike from the meal. To further lower the glycemic load, you may switch from white rice to black, red, or brown rice, which contain more fiber. Because these whole grain rice varieties taste different from white rice, give yourself time to adjust. You can start by splitting your portion of rice between white and brown. You may also find you enjoy substituting farro or millet for rice. Other whole grains that may be substituted include quinoa, bulgur wheat, wheat berries, or barley.

Cooking Grains

The Oldways Whole Grain Council provides some excellent suggestions on how to cook ancient grains on their website, oldwayspt.org. Buckwheat, bulgur, wheat, oats, millet, farro, quinoa, brown rice, and sorghum all take under thirty minutes to prepare. Barley, rye, spelt berries, wheat berries, and wild rice all take forty-five to sixty minutes. Presoaking the grains for a few hours earlier in the day makes the actual cooking time go even faster. You can presoak grains while you are at work, and then cook them quickly for dinner. After cooking, they can keep for the better part of a week in the refrigerator, and you can pull them out to make a bowl with roasted vegetables and tahini sauce, or you can toss them into a soup. Prepare extra grains to freeze or incorporate them into other meals.

The best way to eat grains is to buy them whole, like farro, rolled oats, millet, or quinoa, and cook them at home yourself. Products containing some whole grains will frequently have a whole grain stamp on the label. However, foods like cereals and breads are not typically all whole grain. They frequently contain refined grains combined with whole grains.

Culinary Spotlight: Batch Cooking and Homemade Freezer Meals

Whole grains are perfect for batch cooking, which means doubling the recipe so you can repurpose extra portions for different dishes later in the week. Some ancient grains take longer to cook, so batch cooking can save time in the long run. Extra servings of grains can be stored fresh in the refrigerator to use for multiple meals, or frozen for use in a few weeks or months.

Making your own frozen dinners simply means you've frozen a few extra portions of a meal you spent so much loving care to create, so you can pull it out and enjoy it again in the future on a busy weeknight. You can bet it will be much better than any frozen entrée you would otherwise buy. Just be sure to have a good marker and some blue tape available so you can label what you froze and when you froze it!

Cooking Oats

A few words about oats. Oats are an easy grain for most folks to eat a few times a week. They have so many health benefits and serve as a blank canvas for meals. They are packed with vitamins and minerals, including thiamine, magnesium, manganese, phosphorus, zinc, selenium, and iron. They contain their own type of antioxidants called avenanthramides, as well as soluble and insoluble fiber, which are good for the gut. By adding nuts, nut butter, soy milk, fruits, or vegetables to oats, you reduce the glycemic index of the meal and up its creaminess, sweetness, crunch, and overall comfort factor.

Most people have had oatmeal. The way the oats are prepared will affect their nutritional value. Steel-cut oats, also known as Irish oatmeal, retain the most nutrients. If oats are milled or rolled, they have been stripped of some of their health benefits to allow for quicker cooking. Take the slow road for higher nutrition density. Steel-cut oats may take twenty to thirty minutes to cook, but you can speed this up by soaking the oats the night before.

Overnight Oats (V, VG, GF, DF)

Add 1/2 cup of soy milk and 1/4 cup of steel-cut or rolled oats to a mason jar along with a pinch of salt. Stir well and refrigerate overnight. In the morning, add extra liquid for desired consistency. Heat in the microwave for 30 seconds to warm. Top with fruit, nuts, unsweetened coconut, or nut butter for an indulgent, easy breakfast.

Nutritional Spotlight: Magnesium and Zinc

Magnesium and zinc are two minerals that have been shown to benefit fertility. Magnesium is a mineral found in whole grains, avocados, nuts, and seeds. It helps with cell signaling and energy production, reduces risk for migraines, helps with vitamin D absorption, and helps to prevent chronic diseases such as hypertension and diabetes. Higher miscarriage rate has been observed in women with low magnesium levels.

Zinc is abundant in legumes, shellfish, meat, dairy, and whole grains. It is a key nutrient for male reproductive health; it is involved in enzyme pathways needed for DNA and RNA production, which is vital for spermatogenesis. Zinc is essential for normal functioning of hypothalamic pituitary ovarian (HPO) axis. Low zinc levels can result in low testosterone levels for men.

Stuffed Acorn Squash (V, VG, DF)*

Prep time: 20 minutes
Cook time: 55 minutes
Total time: 75 minutes

Yield: 4 servings

2 medium acorn squash
3 tablespoons extra-virgin
    olive oil, divided
Salt and pepper
¾ cup farro, uncooked
2½ cups vegetable broth
4 ounces tempeh, tofu, or
    vegetarian sausage, cut
    into 1 × ½ inch pieces
1 medium onion, peeled and
    chopped
4 garlic cloves, peeled and
    minced
½ cup chopped celery
½ cup chopped mushrooms
1 tablespoon mixed dried
    Italian herbs (basil,
    thyme, oregano)
¼ cup chopped fresh parsley
⅓ cup chopped nuts (pecans,
    walnuts, or almonds)
¼ cup grated Parmesan
    cheese (optional for
    topping)

Stuffed squash is such a savory treat. Typically available through the fall and winter, squash can be an easy weeknight meal or dressed up for a fancy occasion. This recipe takes a little more time to cook, but it is worthy of a date night with a special someone or a holiday main course. Farro, a hearty ancient grain, has been so popular in our classes that we had to create more ways to enjoy it. Also called "emmer farro," farro has a nutty, toothy texture and is a great source of fiber, protein, and iron. Feel free to substitute any other grain if farro doesn't work for you. We think quinoa would also be great. You can cook the grain in water if you do not have vegetable broth. Acorn squash is just so pretty, and is a good source of magnesium, potassium, manganese, and vitamin C. We love how the tastes and textures cozy up together!

1. Preheat the oven to 400°F. Rinse the squash and microwave whole for 1 minute. Let cool slightly, cut in half, and scoop out the seeds. Brush with olive oil. Season with salt and pepper.

2. Place the squash cut-side down on a baking sheet and roast for 30 to 35 minutes, until a fork can easily pierce the skin. Let cool slightly.

3. While the squash is roasting, prepare the farro stuffing. Rinse the farro, then

combine the farro, vegetable broth, and a teaspoon of salt in a medium saucepan. Bring to a boil over high heat. Cover, reduce heat to medium-low, and simmer until the farro is tender and toothy, about 25 to 35 minutes.

4. Add 2 tablespoons of oil to a large skillet over medium heat. Sauté the tempeh, tofu, or vegetarian sausage until browned, about 3 to 4 minutes. Add onions, garlic, celery, mushrooms, and a pinch of salt, and sauté until the vegetables have softened, about 5 to 6 minutes. Add the dried seasonings.

5. Add the cooked farro stuffing, chopped parsley, and chopped nuts to the skillet, stirring to combine. Season the stuffing with salt to taste.

6. Spoon the farro stuffing into the acorn squash halves on the baking sheet. Optionally, sprinkle the top with Parmesan or vegan cheese.

7. Switch the oven to broil and broil the squash until the tops are golden and the filling is warmed, about 2 minutes.

---

*Vegan and dairy free if vegan Parmesan cheese is used.

Grain Bowls: A Simple Formula

Grain bowls are a staple for us and are usually a mish-mash of what we have on hand. Just combine five simple ingredients: a grain, a leafy green, a vegetable, a protein, and a drizzle of a topping. And there you have it!

Bowls can be a great option for breakfast, lunch, or dinner. Because components are endlessly variable, you can just pick a theme and run with it! Vegetables can be raw, roasted, or steamed. The protein could be chickpeas, black beans, lentils, grilled tofu, or chicken. Grains can be whatever you have on hand. We frequently use farro or quinoa. Add a handful of nuts, seeds, herbs, or dried seaweed for some crunch, and a punchy vinaigrette or creamy topping, and you're good to go!

Sweet Potato Lentil Bowl (V, VG, DF, GF)

Prep time: 10 minutes
Cook time: 35 minutes
Total time: 45 minutes

Yield: 4 servings

For the vegetables:

2 small or 1 medium sweet
   potato, diced into 1-inch
   pieces
1 bunch kale, leaves
   removed from stems,
   about 2 cups
2 tablespoons extra-virgin
   olive oil
Salt

For the lentils:

1½ cups water
½ cup black beluga lentils
   or French green lentils
   (dried)
1 teaspoon garlic powder
½ teaspoon ground
   coriander
½ teaspoon cumin
Salt
1 tablespoon lemon juice
1 teaspoon extra-virgin olive
   oil

Layering lentils, sweet potato, and greens is so easy and delicious. You can sub another root vegetable for the sweet potato, such as carrots, parsnips, or turnips. For the greens, choose a hardy leaf like kale, beet greens, or chard. Feel free to substitute a vegetable or grain that you haven't tried before. It's all flexible! Lemony tahini dressing brings it all together.

1. Rinse the lentils. In a medium pot, combine water, lentils, garlic powder, coriander, cumin, and a pinch of salt. Bring to a boil. Reduce heat to maintain a simmer and cook until tender, 25 to 30 minutes.

2. While the lentils are cooking, rinse the quinoa in a fine mesh strainer. Add the rinsed quinoa to a medium pot with 2 cups of water and a pinch of salt. Bring to a boil on high, then turn down the heat to medium-low. Cover the pot and simmer for about 15 minutes.

3. Steam the diced sweet potato (on the stovetop or in the microwave), for about 5 to 6 minutes, until fork-tender. Let cool.

4. Rinse and dry the kale leaves. Roughly chop or rip the leaves. In a large mixing bowl, massage the kale and a pinch of salt with your hands to soften the leaves.

5. Once most of the water has been absorbed from the quinoa, the germ will

For the quinoa:

1 cup quinoa

2 cups water

Salt

For the dressing:

⅓ cup tahini (sesame seed
   paste)

2 garlic cloves, peeled and
   minced

1 tablespoon extra-virgin
   olive oil

3 tablespoons lemon juice

2 to 4 tablespoons hot water

Garnish (optional):

Cilantro or chives, chopped

have sprouted. Turn off the heat and fluff
with a fork. Leave covered for another 5
minutes.

6. Continue simmering the lentils until the
   liquid reduces slightly, about 5 minutes or
   more. Drain any excess liquid. Stir in the
   lemon juice and olive oil.

7. Combine tahini dressing ingredients in a
   bowl using a whisk or a blender. Slowly
   add water to thin as desired.

8. Assemble bowls with a handful of kale,
   ½ cup of lentils, ½ cup of quinoa, and
   ½ cup of sweet potatoes. Drizzle with the
   tahini dressing. Salt to taste.

9. Garnish with the chopped cilantro or
   chives.

Kitchen Tip: Double this recipe for additional meals during the week.

Jodie's Story

Jodie was thirty-three and felt her biological clock ticking. She and Nick had always planned to have children, but with Nick five years younger than Jodie, they needed to find the right time. They tried to get pregnant for about a year without success and knew it was time to schedule a fertility appointment. After their initial evaluations, they found that Jodie had no issues, but Nick did. Nick had been taking testosterone and had been unaware that it could drastically reduce his sperm production. He was prescribed a medicine to improve his very low sperm count. He needed to improve it tenfold, but it didn't happen, so low-tech therapy would not be an option; they would need IVF. Jodie had to lower her BMI to meet clinic parameters for IVF. So now the pressure was on. They were advised to see a fertility dietitian.

When Jodie and Nick first met with Judy, they were drinking a processed, ready-made liquid meal replacement, Soylent, in an effort to try to eat healthier. They were also eating fast food almost every night. McDonalds, Taco Bell, Pizza Hut, and Asian takeout made up their dinner fare.

Judy guided them and developed a realistic plan with them, focusing on more nutrient-dense, minimally processed prepared frozen or fresh meals instead of fast food and liquid meal replacements. Life was busy for them, so Judy suggested they stick with some of the ready-made meals and add additional vegetables. Jodie loved the simplicity and felt it was doable. "I didn't feel like I was on a diet!" she said.

Jodie also appreciated learning about the benefits of increasing her physical activity to improve her IVF success rate and agreed to add more movement into her routine. Being a scientist, she was happy Judy could provide research that showed the link between nutrition and physical activity and better IVF outcomes. We joked that Jodie took this project on as an engineer; that was her world. She was on board.

It was easy for Jodie to bring frozen meals to work and pick up a large salad from her local café. She also built more walking into her day. She walked to the bus and to on-campus meetings. All her one-on-one meetings with coworkers became walking meetings. She really loved the routine and felt so much healthier. They stuck to this plan for six months with no calorie counting, just focusing on adding in vegetables and Jodie being as healthy as possible. Before long, she made the BMI cutoff and her IVF retrieval resulted in three excellent embryos. About nine months later, Jodie and Nick delivered a healthy baby girl. Jodie's pregnancy was textbook normal, and her OB never talked about weight.

_____

Takeaways

1. Refined, enriched, and fortified are words to describe processed grains that have had the bran and the germ removed (the fiber is gone). These grains are considered simple carbohydrates and have a higher glycemic index.

2. Whole grains are nutrient-dense, complex carbohydrates containing the bran, the germ, and the endosperm. Containing more fiber and nutrients than simple carbohydrates, they are digested more slowly and are good for gut health. They have a lower glycemic index.

3. Whole grains include many ancient grains. Gluten-containing whole grains include farro and wheat berries. Non-gluten whole grains include quinoa and brown rice.

4. Batch cooking can save time by doubling staple preparations for use in multiple recipes.

5. Magnesium and zinc are important minerals to support fertility.

6. Ultra-processed foods go through chemical processing, lack fiber, and cause inflammation. They are frequently high glycemic. These attributes can negatively impact fertility.

Sample SMART Goals

1. Try a new grain like wheat berries, farro, or quinoa this week.
2. When eating simple carbs, combine them with a protein like a nut butter or hummus.
3. Cook a double batch recipe of grains. Meal plan two recipes that use that grain within five days.
4. Make a Grain bowl using five components: a grain, a green, a legume, a vegetable, and a dressing.
5. Don't keep junk food in the house, or keep it "out of sight, out of mind."

Chapter 5

Lusty Legumes

Test Your Knowledge

Beans are full of carbohydrates. True/False

*Tofu is safe when I'm trying to get pregnant.** True/False

Why are legumes lusty? Because they are bursting with good health and pack a crazy amount of nutrition in a small package. Beans and lentils are high in fiber, carbohydrates, vitamins, and minerals, not to mention 30 percent protein! One serving of lentils, about half a cup, provides 7 to 9 grams of fiber, 8 grams of protein, 20 grams of carbohydrates, and 1 gram of fat. We hope you can learn to love them as much as we do.

There are three subtypes of legumes: dried, fresh, and oilseed. The first type, dried seeds, are commonly known as pulses, or beans and lentils. Included in the dried family are chickpeas, black beans, pinto beans, cannellini beans, navy beans, lentils, dried split peas, black-eyed peas, mung beans, and

---

* True. Beans are a great source of sustained energy because Mother Nature includes protein, carbohydrates, fiber, vitamins, and minerals to decrease the time their energy enters our bloodstream. They help us to feel satisfied longer and help to balance our insulin and glucose levels.

** True. Soy foods, including tofu, edamame, tempeh, and soy milk, are fertility-promoting and perfectly safe to eat while trying to conceive.

kidney beans. The pulse category also includes all types of lentils including red, green, brown, French, Puy, black beluga, chana dal, urad dal, and moong dal, to name a few. Many pulses will be available at your local grocery store, while other specialty beans and lentils may be purchased in a specialty store or ordered online. Dried pulses are an easily seasoned, inexpensive staple consumed by a large percentage of the global population on a daily basis.

The second subcategory of legumes is one that we frequently associate with vegetables: peas. Peas are actually classified as a legume, not a vegetable. They contain more protein than most vegetables. In fact, pea protein is sometimes isolated and used as a plant-based protein powder.[1] Peas come wrapped in a pod. Some peas require shelling prior to eating, like English peas and fava beans. Others do not, such as sugar snap peas, snow peas, and snap beans, all of which have edible pods. There are many specialty subtypes as well, which you can grow in your garden. Of course, fresh peas are not that different from dried and split peas, other than being fresh.

The third subcategory of legumes, oilseed legumes, includes soybeans and peanuts. Compared to the non-oilseed legumes (dry pulses and fresh peas), the oilseed legumes have higher fat content and lower fiber. Whole soybeans, known as edamame, are a delicious, healthful snack. Tempeh, tofu, and unsweetened soy milk are excellent sources of complete protein and carbohydrates. And don't forget that fabulous fiber.

The protein content in soybeans is higher than other plants, and soy contains all the essential amino acids, similar to animal protein. The oligosaccharide carbohydrate found in soy is not digested well by our small intestine but is enjoyed greatly by the bacteria in our colon, making them a prebiotic. The fat in soybeans consists of the healthy omega-6 and omega-3 polyunsaturated fatty acids. Soybeans are also high in potassium and iron.

Soy is a common agricultural crop that is frequently processed into an isolate. This chemically processed food additive, known as soy protein isolate, is frequently added to protein bars and powders. Although soy protein isolate is high in protein, it has had many nutrients removed, including most of the fiber and fat. Choosing whole-food soybeans is always preferable for overall nutrient density over an isolated soy nutrient.

Health Benefits

Legumes are a good source of fiber, B vitamins, iron, copper, magnesium, zinc, and phosphorus. They can lower the risk of hypertension, diabetes, stroke, and heart disease.[2] The fiber also serves as a prebiotic for the gut microbiome and improves insulin sensitivity. Pulses, along with vegetables, can also improve mental health. The National Health and Nutrition Examination Survey cohort (NHANES) showed that people who ate more fiber experienced a decrease in depression.[3]

Legumes are low glycemic and eating them can result in lower average glucose levels. A study of 121 subjects with type 2 diabetes demonstrated that the group randomized to consume at least one cup of legumes daily had a decrease in their hemoglobin A1C levels by a half a percent compared to those who just consumed wheat fiber.[4] The polyphenols in beans improve blood glucose and cholesterol levels, are anti-inflammatory, and are good for cardiometabolic health.[5] Additional studies have shown that legumes can also aid in losing weight. In 2016, a meta-analysis looked at twenty-one different trials with more than 940 participants. There was a small but significant weight reduction for the groups that incorporated pulses into their diets compared to those who did not.[6] This was observed even when calories were not restricted. Soluble fiber in beans decreases gastric emptying and the protein in beans increases secretion of some satiety hormones. Both effects lead to a prolonged sense of fullness and lower rise in blood sugar after eating.

Soy has some additional nutritional benefits. The isoflavones in soy can act as estrogenic polyphenols, or phytoestrogens, and selective estrogen receptor modulators (SERM), all of which means they act like estrogen but are derived from plants. The most common soy isoflavones are genistein and daidzein. By binding to the estrogen receptor, they can have estrogen-promoting or estrogen-blocking effects. In many Asian countries, the average soy consumption far exceeds average consumption in the United States, and it does not create a hormonal imbalance with excess of estrogen. In fact, soy consumption has been shown to reduce mortality for those with a history of breast cancer in North America.[7] In another study, consumption of soy isoflavones in women following a diagnosis of breast cancer showed a reduced risk of breast cancer recurrence and a reduced risk of mortality from breast cancer.[8]

Pulses, like fruits, vegetables, and whole grains, are an excellent source of fiber. Compared to other foods, vegetables and pulses have the highest fiber content by far. If people focused on meeting their fiber needs, most would meet more of their overall nutritional needs.[9] Many people eating a plant-based diet easily consume more than 60 grams of fiber per day. Depending on your body size, you may want to aim for 40 to 60 grams of fiber and 50 to 70 grams of protein per day. Over 90 percent of the population in the United States gets more protein than they need, but not enough fiber.

In the following table, we compare the fiber, fat, and protein content of a typical serving size of different foods. The legumes win for having the best combination of fiber and protein.[10] Whole grains and nuts are pretty good, but the animal sources contain no fiber.

Comparing Fiber, Protein, and Fat in Foods

Foods per serving size	Dietary fiber, grams	Protein, grams	Fat, grams
Almonds (12 almonds)	2.2	3.0	7.5
Broccoli (1 cup cooked)	3.0	3.0	0
Brown rice (½ cup cooked)	2.5	5.0	0.8
Carrots, sliced (1 cup cooked)	4.7	1.0	0
Chicken breast (½ medium breast)	0	29.0	7.8
Chickpeas (½ cup cooked)	7.0	7.0	1.0
Edamame (½ cup cooked)	4.0	9.0	4.0
Egg (1 large)	0	6.3	5.0
Lentils (½ cup cooked)	9.0	8.5	0.3
Quinoa (½ cup cooked)	3.0	5.0	2.0
Raspberries (1 cup)	8.0	1.5	0.8
Salmon (3 ounces, cooked)	0	17.0	9.2

Foods per serving size	Dietary fiber, grams	Protein, grams	Fat, grams
Split peas (½ cup cooked)	4.0	4.0	0.4
Tofu, firm (¼ package)	1.0	13.0	8.0

Source: U.S. Department of Agriculture, Agricultural Research Service, FoodData Central (usda.gov) 2019, and manufacturer labels

Fertility Benefits

Legumes are part of a fertility-promoting diet, along with fruits, vegetables, whole grains, and fish.[11] Soy is known to be especially fertility promoting, particularly in its whole or minimally processed forms. In fact, higher phytoestrogen levels (from consumption of soy) have been associated with shorter time to pregnancy for women[12] and higher pregnancy rates with IVF.[13] The EARTH study found individuals undergoing IVF treatment who consumed soy had the additional benefit of reducing endocrine disruptors and improved successful IVF births.[14] In another study, women with a higher urinary concentration of lignans, one of the phytoestrogens found in soy and whole grains, demonstrated a shorter time to pregnancy.[15]

A few studies have found soy benefited women with PCOS. One study looked at the effect of soy on metabolic parameters. Sixty women with PCOS were randomized to either eat a diet with 35 percent of their protein coming from soy, 35 percent from animal protein, and 30 percent from plant protein, or 70 percent from animal protein and 30 percent from plant protein. The group following the diet with soy experienced lowered fasting glucose and insulin resistance, as well as lower testosterone and triglyceride levels.[16] Another pilot study compared the effect of increased intake of soy milk for three days on the microbiota (bacteria in our gut) in women with PCOS compared to those without PCOS.[17] After the intervention, there was a higher number of species of gut bacteria, better glucose metabolism, and improved androgen (another type of sex hormone) levels in women with PCOS. No difference was observed in the control group.

We believe if you try a few of our recipes you will easily eat more legumes every week. They are inexpensive and add texture and flavor to your meals. For everyone following a plant-forward diet, they are one of the main fiber and protein staples.

Cooking Legumes

Legumes can be cooked ahead of time, drained, and stored in the refrigerator. When you are shopping for dried beans, look for whole beans with bright colors and minimal cracked or broken beans. Younger dried beans have a shine to them, while older beans look dull. Older beans will continue to dry out and require longer cooking times. They should be stored in a dark, dry location in a tightly sealed bag or glass jar. We prefer using dried beans and soaking for an hour or overnight. These will taste better than canned beans and produce less gas when digested. But canned beans can be a time saver in a pinch, and we definitely have canned or boxed beans in our pantry. If using canned beans, drain and rinse the liquid to reduce some of the added sodium.

Before cooking, look through your beans and discard any small stones or broken or shriveled beans. Then, ideally, soak your beans for a minimum of one hour or up to a day, which will help to rehydrate them and lower the cooking time. Cover the beans with plenty of cold water, using about three to four times as much water as beans. Soaking will also help to remove some of the indigestible sugars associated with future gassiness from consuming beans. Beans that have been soaked overnight have the shortest cooking time, but for a quick soak, bring beans to a boil for two to three minutes, then let cool for one hour. Skim off any foam and skins that may have risen to the surface. Always be sure to drain and rinse your soaked beans and add lots of fresh cold water before cooking. Some soaked beans will lose a little color and a few nutrients, but we think the trade-off in shortened cooking time is worth it. Lentils and dried split peas are small enough that they do not require presoaking.

After soaking most legumes, you're ready to cook them. In a regular pot on the stove, bring beans to a boil and then reduce to a simmer for the recommended cooking time. Boiling is too rough and will split the skins. Smaller legumes cook faster. Lentils cook in ten to forty minutes and do not require any soaking time. Others, like chickpeas and kidney beans, are larger and take about two hours to cook.

Cooking times will vary based on the age and storage condition of the beans, so check them occasionally if you are cooking on a stovetop. Salt is best added to the beans or lentils about three quarters of the way through the cooking time. When beans are done, they should be intact, creamy, and tender, but not mushy. Split peas and lentils may be cooked until they break down if a more puréed consistency is desired. It is a good idea to reserve some of the cooking liquid from beans as a stock to use with your intended dish if making a soup or stew.

When cooking chickpeas, save some of the cooking liquid for added flavor rather than water. The liquid is known as "aquafaba" and has binding properties similar to eggs. Add a little salt, and it is a savory broth for sipping. When you make hummus, the cooking liquid from the chickpeas can be used when blending to the desired consistency.

You can speed up the cooking process dramatically by using a pressure cooker or Instant Pot. Cooking under pressure can reduce cooking times by another 30 to 70 percent. Be sure to read the directions for safe use of your equipment. It is very important to never open the lid while pressure is still built up or serious injuries can occur. When using a pressure cooker, never fill the pot more than two thirds full. A pound of dried beans in the Instant Pot can yield the equivalent of four cans of beans in just one hour. They will taste fresh and have no slime, and you can freeze the extra beans in silicone bags for future recipes. The only disadvantage of cooking under pressure is that you cannot monitor the progress as the cooking occurs, so you need to know how long to cook the beans before turning off the heat. Salt and season the beans later, however you choose to use them, if they have been cooked under pressure.

Feeling Gassy?

If you get gassy and uncomfortable after eating beans, you can try taking Beano or Bean-zyme, which is also known as alpha-1-galacto-sidase, before your meal. You can try adding a piece of kombu seaweed when you are cooking beans, which also contains alpha-1-galactosi-dase, to help reduce raffinose, an undigestible sugar containing galactose, glucose, and fructose.

Eating fermented foods more regularly will also boost the number of good bacteria in the gut and reduce gas. Fermented foods like kimchi or sauerkraut are "double bonus" foods. They function as both prebiotics and probiotics: prebiotics because they contain fiber from cabbage and other vegetables that the gut bacteria get to digest, and probiotics because they are flush with their own bacteria, which have multiplied during the fermentation process. Yogurt and kefir are fermented forms of dairy that also contain bacteria such as Lactobacillus, Bifidobacterium, and other species which promote gut health. Look for the phrase "live active cultures" on the label to ensure they are probiotic.

Seasoning Legumes

Legumes can be seasoned many different ways. They are used all over the world, and depending on your preference, you can enjoy them in Mediterranean, Asian, Mexican, African, and Central, North, or South American dishes. They combine well with lemon or yogurt, as well as spices such as cumin, coriander, turmeric, or cayenne. Try mixing some lentils with olive oil, garlic, lemon juice, parsley, salt, and pepper, adding some feta, olives, and cherry tomatoes, and serving over some fresh leafy greens to make an easy Mediterranean salad. Legumes can be used in vegetarian recipes or combined with small amounts of animal protein. They can be combined with a whole grain to make a meal complete with all the essential amino acids. They make a great addition to salads, soups, and bowls for a nutrient-packed lunch or dinner.

Get to Know Dal

Dal is an uncomplicated, delicious stew of lentils and spices. Many people in India, Nepal, and around the world eat dal every day. An easy variety involves boiling 1 cup of red lentils, 3 cups of water, 1/2 teaspoon of turmeric, and one teaspoon of salt for about 10 to 12 minutes until thick and soft. In a separate small skillet, sauté two or three cloves of finely chopped garlic, 1/2 teaspoon of finely chopped ginger, 1/2 teaspoon of ground cumin, and a small green chili or 1/2 teaspoon of red pepper flakes in a tablespoon of ghee or a neutral oil for about a minute. When fragrant, add the contents of the skillet into the cooked lentils, and add salt to taste. Serve over brown rice or another whole grain and garnish with some chopped cilantro. Quick, savory, and satisfying!

Culinary Spotlight: Cooking on a Budget

Beans and lentils lend themselves to cooking on a budget. Buying dry pulses can even be less expensive than canned. In stores or online, these can easily be purchased and stored in your pantry. A serving of beans that you soak and cook at home may cost less than a dollar. Have an organized pantry of pulses and grains so you can pull together a weeknight meal quickly. Store pulses and grains in clear, labeled containers to easily identify them.

Nutritional Spotlight: Iron

Iron is a trace mineral required for our bodies in small quantities. Iron is found in plants and animals and is important for the production of hemoglobin, which carries oxygen in our blood. Iron deficiency can result from heavy menstrual periods or inadequate dietary consumption, leading to anemia and fatigue. It is especially important to have enough iron and a normal red blood cell count when preparing for pregnancy, since during pregnancy the blood volume in your body greatly expands. Iron is also important for the function of myoglobin in muscles and in other cells for energy metabolism. It is essential for egg development in a growing follicle.

There are two types of iron, heme iron and nonheme iron. Heme iron can be found in shellfish, poultry, beef, and organ meats such as liver. It can also be found in "enriched" foods that are iron-fortified such as cereals or grains. Nonheme iron is found in legumes, mushrooms, and dark green leafy vegetables, nutritional yeast, and dried fruit. Intake of vitamin C from citrus, berries, tomatoes, or broccoli can enhance the absorption of nonheme iron. Also, combining a small amount of heme iron can enhance the bioavailability of nonheme iron. Other foods and beverages—including phytates such as unprocessed grains and polyphenols such as coffee, tea, spinach, and red wine—contain compounds called chelators that can decrease the absorption of iron.

The recommended iron intake is 18 milligrams a day for women and 8 milligrams a day for men. Some individuals consuming a plant-based diet may have difficulty reaching the recommended intake with food alone and may require iron supplementation. This can be taken separately or as part of a multivitamin. Most people who menstruate and are trying to conceive should look for a prenatal vitamin that contains iron. The easiest way to make sure you do not have iron-deficiency anemia is to check your complete blood count (CBC) and ferritin level. In one study, women at risk for iron deficiency due to heavy menses or a short menstrual interval had increased pregnancy rates when they increased the intake of nonheme iron from their diet and iron supplements.[18]

Split Pea Soup (V, VG, DF)

Prep time: 10 minutes
Cook time: 40 minutes
Total time: 50 minutes

Yield: 6 to 8 servings

1 tablespoon extra-virgin
   olive oil
2 cups diced onions
1½ cups diced carrots
1½ cups diced celery
   (optional to include
   celery tops)
Salt, as needed
2 cups dried split peas
6 cups vegetable broth
3 bay leaves
1 teaspoon dried thyme
2 to 3 tablespoons white
   miso paste (optional)
Chives to garnish (optional)

Soup's on! Velvety split pea soup in under an hour with a secret ingredient, miso, that adds umami to this classic soup. Peas, as a legume, are a protein powerhouse. They are high in carbohydrates, fiber, and vitamins A and K. They also provide lots of polyphenols, which are good antioxidants for fertility. You may recognize the slowly sautéed combination of onions, carrots, and celery as the classic mirepoix blend, which gives a sweet flavor to this soup. Miso paste comes from fermented soybeans, another legume; the soybeans are combined with rice koji or barley koji for fermentation. The barley koji is not gluten free, for those who need to avoid gluten. We prefer white miso for this soup, which is more mellow and slightly sweeter and less salty than the red variety. To preserve its lovely aroma, miso should not be boiled, but added to the end of the soup once the heat is off. Miso can add saltiness to the dish, so taste before adding any extra salt. If you prefer your split pea soup even creamier, you can blend it after it has cooled slightly.

1. In a 6-quart pot over medium heat, add olive oil, onions, carrots, celery, and a pinch of salt. Sauté 5 to 6 minutes over medium-low heat until the vegetables start to soften but do not brown.
2. Rinse the split peas. Add the broth and peas to the pot with a generous pinch of

salt, the bay leaves, and the thyme, and bring to a boil. Reduce heat to a simmer, cover, and continue to cook.

3. Simmer for 30 minutes with occasional stirring until the peas are very soft and the soup becomes creamy when stirred.

4. Discard the bay leaves.

5. Thin 2 to 3 tablespoons of miso in warm water and whisk to blend, then add to the soup. Salt to taste.

6. Garnish with finely chopped chives.

Stir-Fried Cabbage and Tofu (V, VG, DF, GF)

Prep time: 10 minutes

Cook time: 10 minutes

Total time: 20 minutes

Yield: 4 servings

1 (14-ounce) package firm or extra-firm tofu

Salt

½ head of Napa cabbage (or other greens of your choice), quartered, cored, and cut into 2-inch pieces

2 tablespoons neutral oil, such as avocado or canola

½ teaspoon red pepper flakes (optional)

2 to 3 garlic cloves, peeled and minced

Splash of tamari*

2 tablespoons water

Splash of rice vinegar (optional)

½ teaspoon sugar (optional)

2 tablespoons chopped green onions

Many home cooks stir-fry a single vegetable, such as a leafy green, green beans, or broccoli, and make it delicious. This recipe combines Napa cabbage, green cabbage, bok choy, mustard greens, or any single leafy green with garlic and tamari for a flavorful dish. We add tofu for extra protein. Any of these stir-fried greens can be served with brown rice or noodles.

1. Open the tofu package and drain. Press the tofu block by putting it between two plates for 5 minutes.

2. Dry the tofu with paper towels and cut into 1-inch cubes. Sprinkle tofu with a pinch of salt and toss in a mixing bowl.

3. In a mixing bowl, massage the cabbage or other greens lightly with a pinch of salt to separate and soften the leaves.

4. Add the neutral oil to a wok or large skillet and heat on high heat until shimmering, less than one minute.

5. Toss the red pepper flakes into the wok followed by the tofu cubes 30 seconds later and stir-fry for 5 to 8 minutes until the tofu is golden brown on a few sides. Remove the tofu and place on a plate.

6. Add the garlic to the skillet and toss for 30 seconds, followed by the cabbage or other leafy greens. Stir-fry for about 3 to 5 minutes until the greens are slightly charred. Be sure not to overload the pan;

you may have to stir-fry the cabbage in two batches.

7. Add the tofu and mix. Sprinkle the sides of the pan with tamari and water. Stir and taste. Add more soy sauce as desired to taste.

8. For optional sweet and sour flavoring, add rice vinegar and a sprinkle of sugar.

9. Garnish with green onions.

---

*The use of tamari instead of soy sauce in this recipe keeps it gluten free. Soy sauce and tamari are both produced from fermented soybeans and add a salty, umami flavor. Soy sauce is made from soy and wheat. If you have celiac disease or sensitivity to gluten, stick to tamari which is made from 100 percent soy.

Kristina's Story

Kristina knew from a very early age that she wanted to be a mom. So, when she got married at twenty-two, she stopped oral contraceptives. A few months later, she skipped a menstrual cycle and did a pregnancy test, but it was negative. "What is going on with my body?" she wondered. She learned from her doctor at the time that she had PCOS. When Kristina and her husband came in to see Dr. Thyer, they talked about PCOS, how it could cause infertility, and how they could treat it. They let her know that they didn't want to be too aggressive, so they started with some basic testing. Her husband's sperm count was good, and her fallopian tubes were open. Her menstrual cycles had been getting progressively longer and longer, forty days, then fifty or more. She was not ovulating but wanted to try a natural approach first.

Dr. Thyer recommended she meet with Judy Simon, focus on lifestyle changes to start, and join the Food for Fertility class. She was hesitant to meet with a nutritionist. "You know there are things you're not supposed to do, like eat fast food, and I feel like going into it, they're going to give me a list of things that I already know I'm not supposed to do, and it's going to make me feel guilty."

But thankfully, that wasn't the case. "That's one thing that surprised me," Kristina recalled, "I don't think I've ever heard Judy say, 'Don't eat something.' She'd always say, 'Okay, you're eating that, that's fine. How about you think about adding something healthier into your diet?' It was such a refreshing way of looking at lifestyle changes. There was no condemnation or guilt with it. At the very least, I could add in these new foods. There were things that I was introduced to that I never would have tried on my own. I don't know what they are, and I don't know what they taste like." Kristina had a natural curiosity about new foods and was developing into a competent eater.

I asked what some of her new foods were. "Shallots—now I cook with these, not like it's something huge. Quinoa, never had quinoa, never knew what it was. Edamame is the other thing. I'd never heard of it. We tried it fresh, and I loved it! We put it in a stir-fry, and it was really yummy!" She appreciated the fact that there was never anything wrong with anything she did. No guilt, only encouragement.

Kristina and her husband had been trying for about a year without success. To avoid seeing people at church over Mother's Day, they decided to plan a weekend getaway on one of the neighboring islands off the coast of northern Washington. She wanted to relax, go hiking, and enjoy some nice meals and a few drinks. She figured she should take a pregnancy test since she had some spotting, but her period hadn't started. There was a faint line on the test. Her husband said it was probably nothing, to just take another one. Same thing, slight line. "We ended up buying three more tests, and when I saw the one that actually tells you with words, 'pregnant,' I finally believed I was pregnant!"

Takeaways

1. Legumes include beans, lentils, peas, and soybeans. They are a great source of fiber and protein.
2. Diets lacking fiber can damage the gut microbiome and lead to dysbiosis and inflammation. Include lots of legumes and vegetables in your diet to protect the gut. Food from animal sources does not contain fiber.
3. Check your complete blood count and ferritin level. Supplement iron if your ferritin level is low or if you have iron-deficiency anemia.

Sample SMART Goals

1. Compare dried, soaked, and cooked beans to canned beans for taste.
2. Try a new lentil, bean, or soy recipe this week.
3. Try batch cooking and freezing beans or lentils to save time with a future meal.
4. Once you have slowly increased your fiber intake, aim to eat ½ cup to 1 cup of legumes most days.

Chapter 6

Dairy and Plant Milks

Test Your Knowledge

*Almond milk is the healthiest milk.** True/False

*Dairy is the main source of calcium in our diets.*** True/False

Many people grew up with the common dairy staples, milk and cheese. Cheese is so well loved that the average consumer in the United States eats about forty pounds per year! But, as people get older, milk and cheese can become harder to digest. Cheese is also one of the largest sources of saturated fat.

About half of adults have difficulty digesting dairy products due to the presence of lactose, a sugar contained in milk. The lactase gene, which determines how well your body is able to break down the lactose found in dairy, is expressed during infancy and early childhood, but its expression is reduced

---

* False. Most almond milks are mostly water with very little actual almonds (unless homemade). Other plant milks such as soy or pea offer much more nutrition, including about the same amount of protein as cow's milk.

** False. You can get calcium from almonds, tofu, beans, lentils, nuts, seeds, greens, and black strap molasses. One cup of edamame provides 27 percent of your daily needs.

for some populations in adulthood, making it harder to digest dairy. People who produce less of the lactase enzyme may experience uncomfortable gastrointestinal symptoms when they consume too much dairy. It's worth clarifying that this is due to being unable to digest the lactose found in dairy, and not because dairy causes inflammation. In fact, dairy may have anti-inflammatory benefits. That being said, if you can't tolerate dairy, don't enjoy it, or choose not to consume it, that is okay.

Even with some degree of lactose intolerance, small amounts of dairy may be tolerated by most individuals. Hard cheeses, such as Parmesan, have minimal amounts of lactose and may complement some dishes. Interestingly, yogurt, which contains live cultures of lactobacilli, can usually be consumed in larger amounts without difficulty. Yogurt and kefir are fermented with live cultures and are good for the gut microbiota. But be aware that hidden sugars are added to many brands of yogurt. Look for unsweetened varieties and add your own fruit for sweetness.

A Few Words on Cheese

The world is filled with some amazing cheeses that can complement your cooking. Soft, hard, or somewhere in between, the flavor of cheese is affected by the diet of the animal it came from and their environment. Cheese has a number of nutrients including calcium; vitamins B12, A, and K; and protein. Many varieties contain naturally occurring bacteria that act as probiotics. Cheese can also have a high amount of saturated fat and sodium. For a fertility-promoting diet, we recommend cheese as a condiment and flavor accent, rather than a main ingredient. From a nutrition standpoint, cheese may be enjoyed in moderation as part of a plant-forward diet. For those who do not consume dairy, there are some good plant-based alternatives.

Health Benefits

Nutrients in dairy include protein, calcium, phosphorus, magnesium, vitamin D, vitamin A, and B vitamins. Fermented dairy, like yogurt and kefir, contains probiotics good for gut health. Calcium and vitamin D, which are found in dairy, are needed for bone health. Calcium can come from dairy, but it can come from nondairy foods and drinks as well.

Nutritional Spotlight: Calcium

In addition to bone strength, calcium provides help with blood clotting and nerve transmission. Adequate calcium is recommended for bone health and may reduce the risk of colon cancer, but too much calcium can increase the risk of heart disease, ovarian cancer, and prostate cancer. Although milk contains calcium, not all the calcium in milk can be absorbed. Calcium is better absorbed when combined with vitamin D. Other sources of calcium include dark leafy greens, salmon, soy, beans, and other legumes. Plant milks are frequently supplemented with calcium and other vitamins. The Recommended Dietary Allowance (RDA) for calcium for women and men of reproductive age is 1,000 milligrams daily, with most coming from food.[1]

Fertility Benefits

Full-fat dairy in limited quantities is considered generally beneficial for fertility compared to low-fat dairy. One large observational study showed that women who consume low-fat dairy had an increased risk of ovulatory infertility compared to those who consumed high-fat dairy foods.[2] For men, some studies have shown just the opposite; better sperm parameters were associated with low-fat dairy versus high-fat dairy.[3] The thing to remember about observational studies is that they show an association, but not causation.

In the rest of the medical world, the nutritional benefits of high-fat versus low-fat dairy are debated with regard to long-term health. Based on existing data for women who are trying to conceive, we favor full-fat dairy over low-fat or nonfat dairy. Ideally, this would be a cup of whole-fat Greek yogurt daily, rather than an eight-ounce glass of milk since fermented dairy has additional health benefits for the gut. For men, if sperm factors are a concern, low-fat dairy is preferred.

The data on dairy shows that its health effects are not all positive, however. A cohort from the EARTH study looked at consumption of dairy and found that those who had the highest dairy intake, greater than two cups per day, had the lowest antral follicle counts. The antral follicle count refers to the number of small follicles (fluid-filled sacs) containing eggs. It is used to predict ovarian reserve by acting as a surrogate marker for the overall recruitable pool of eggs any given month.[4] When you are trying to get pregnant, especially when you are using assisted reproductive technologies like IVF, you don't want to lower the number of eggs you may be able to stimulate. So, the current data suggests that consuming no dairy may be neutral, about a cup a day may be beneficial, and two cups a day may be unfavorable.

Nutritional Spotlight: Vitamin D

Vitamin D can be considered both a vitamin (an essential nutrient that facilitates chemical reactions in the body) and a hormone (something manufactured by the body that causes responses in tissues). The metabolite of vitamin D has many important roles in the body. It supports bone health, immune health, brain function, and reproductive health. It is an antioxidant and has anti-inflammatory properties.

A number of studies appear to show better IVF outcomes in patients with normal versus low vitamin D levels,[5] and treating vitamin D deficiency in couples undergoing IVF may lead to better embryo quality and higher pregnancy rates.[6,7] Vitamin D deficiency can be more common in women with PCOS and treating vitamin D deficiency may help to restore normal ovulation and menstrual frequency.[8] Vitamin D supplementation has also been shown to improve IVF outcomes in infertile women with PCOS and insulin resistance.[9] In men, higher vitamin D levels are associated positively with sperm quality.[10] Vitamin D deficiency has been associated with miscarriage, but it is yet to be determined whether treating the deficiency with extra vitamin D reduces miscarriage rate.[11] Treating vitamin D deficiency has been shown to reduce risk of maternal and fetal adverse events.[12]

Unfortunately, there are not great sources of vitamin D in food, though some dairy milk and plant-based milks are fortified with a small amount of vitamin D, about 100 international units (IU) per serving. Rather, vitamin D comes mainly from sun exposure on the skin. Vitamin D deficiency is very common in northern latitudes due to the angle of the sun's rays and less duration of exposure to sunlight, and deficiency can increase susceptibility to infections, cardiovascular disease, and depression.

Depending on where you live, it may be difficult to get enough vitamin D from sunlight or food, so many people take vitamin D supplements. Many multivitamins or prenatal vitamins may have 400 IU of vitamin D. Taking 400 to 2,000 IU of vitamin D3 daily will help many people maintain adequate levels. Some women may need to take higher levels of supplementation year-round to maintain adequate vitamin D levels. If in doubt, ask to have your vitamin D (25-hydroxyvitamin D) checked, and aim to get your level above 30 nanograms per milliliter (ng/mL) while trying to conceive.

Shopping for Dairy

For those who enjoy dairy, look to purchase brands where the cows were not given additional hormones to increase their milk supply. Milk containers will say "no hormones" or "no recombinant bovine growth hormone (rbCH)" or "no recombinant bovine somatotropin (rbST)." They may also highlight qualities like non-GMO, no pesticides, organic, pasture-raised, or grass-fed. Always buy pasteurized milk to decrease the risk of any harmful bacterial consumption from raw dairy. Ideally look for organic, pasteurized, grass-fed milk for the highest nutrient quality. Grass-fed, full-fat milk, and butter will have more omega-3s as well as vitamins E and K, two fat-soluble vitamins important for our health.

Plant-Based Milks

Plant milks are a growing sector of the market as many consumers look for alternatives to dairy. Taste and affordability are the most common drivers of purchase choice. The most common plant-based milks are almond, coconut, soy, and oat. The nutritional content and environmental impact can vary quite a bit between types.

Many plant-based milk varieties now take up a significant portion of the chilled dairy case at the grocery store. Each plant milk has different nutritional benefits and tastes, so feel free to experiment. Plant milks sold in stores are frequently fortified with calcium and vitamin D. They may have algal acid added to boost omega-3 fatty acid levels and improve the mouthfeel. They also frequently contain emulsifiers like lecithin to keep the plant milk from separating and thickeners like guar gum for consistency. They may also contain added sugars, sweeteners, or flavors. Take a look at the label when buying plant milk and try to avoid added sugars or sweeteners. If buying one with just the plant and water, without added emulsifiers, it will need to be shaken to resuspend the settled solids before drinking.

The plant milks with the highest protein content are soy milk and pea protein milk, which contain about 8 grams per cup. Soy milk was one of the first plant milks widely available and is one of the most nutritious, with anti-inflammatory and antioxidant properties from isoflavones. Soy milk may be the best choice for those trying to conceive, as soy has been recognized as contributing to a fertility-promoting diet.[13] It also has the closest nutritional composition to full-fat dairy. Pea protein milk also has high protein, moderate fat, and low carbohydrate content. It is frequently fortified with potassium, calcium, vitamins A and D, and iron. Other nut milks have naturally lower protein content. Sometimes pea protein is added to other commercial plant milks to build up the protein content.

Almond milk has become an increasingly popular plant milk option and has fewer calories than soy milk, but little protein. Its environmental impact is also higher compared with other options: almond trees require more water than other nut trees, and some people, recognizing the scarcity of water in places like California, are looking to other environmentally friendly plant-based alternatives. Oat milk is earth friendly and popular among consumers but contains very little protein. It consists of rolled oats blended with water. It has twice the carbohydrates as almond milk and more fiber. Rice milk also has minimal protein. Coconut milk has more saturated fat than other plant milks and no protein. Hemp milk has an earthy flavor and contains a moderate amount of protein, omega-3 and omega-6 fatty acids, and some iron. It may also be fortified with calcium, vitamin D, phosphorus, vitamin A, and vitamin B12. Flaxseed milk contains omega-3 fatty acids and also has a nutty flavor. Cashew milk is easy to make at home and has lots of fiber and nutrients like magnesium. It has a very neutral taste and, depending on how much water is blended with the presoaked cashews, it can be used as a creamy nondairy base to make a white sauce. Commercial cashew milk has been strained and contains less protein and fiber than the homemade variety. It is typically fortified with vitamins and minerals.

Shopping for Plant Milks

The number of plant-based milk options may feel overwhelming, so we've broken down the data for you. When shopping, look for plant milks to be fortified with calcium. As an added benefit, plant milks may be fortified with vitamin D, iodine, and B vitamins. We've put together the following table that compares the protein, fat, and carbohydrate content of dairy milk and a variety of unsweetened plant-based milks.

Protein, Fat, and Carbohydrate Content in Milk Varieties (per 250 ml)

Milk type (unsweetened)	Protein, grams	Fat, grams	Carbohydrate, grams
Dairy, full fat	8.8	8.8	15.0
Almond	1.3	3.0	1.8
Coconut	0.5	5.0	6.0
Oat	3.0	9.0	15.0
Pea	8	4.5	<1
Rice	0	2.5	27
Soy	9.0	7.0	12.0

Source: U.S. Department of Agriculture, Agricultural Research Service, FoodData Central (usda.gov) 2019, and manufacturer labels

Yogurt and Other Fermented Foods

Fermented foods can improve our health, thanks to the live bacteria they contain.[14] When a food has been fermented, it means the bacteria in it have converted the natural sugars in the food into an acid. Yogurt, kefir, sauerkraut, and kimchi are examples of fermented foods. They have a unique, tangy taste from the presence of lactic acid.

Yogurt, which contains lactobacillus, is beneficial for your gut and a mainstay for a Mediterranean diet.[15] We frequently use full-fat plain yogurt in sauces, dips, and dressings, and also in our recipes to add moisture and some tang. Of course, it can also be used in smoothies and as a stand-alone, topped with berries and nuts. Kefir is yogurt's tangier cousin, a fermented milk drink with higher amounts of probiotics, and is also a rich source of calcium, protein, and B vitamins. You can drink kefir like a smoothie, or enjoy it with some fruit and whole grains. Be sure to read the label to avoid added sugars in both yogurt and kefir.

Most people are familiar with yogurt, but kimchi and sauerkraut may be new to you. Think of them as condiments you keep in jars in the refrigerator and pull out to add a spoonful to a grain bowl or something you are cooking. You can make kimchi scrambled eggs by throwing a tablespoon of kimchi into a skillet followed by an egg and slowly cooking to give your breakfast a savory twist. Or you can make sauerkraut beans by adding a spoonful of sauerkraut into a bowl of brothy cannellini beans, pintos, or black-eyed peas. Not only will you increase the fiber content of your meal, but you'll be gaining the advantage of the probiotic food, which is good for gut health!

Yogurt Fruit Parfait (GF)

Prep time: 10 minutes

Total Time: 10 minutes

Yield: 1 serving

½ to ¾ cup full-fat Greek yogurt

½ cup berries or other fruits, chopped or sliced

¼ cup chopped or sliced nuts (walnuts, almonds, pecans)

Full-fat yogurt is a great source of protein, probiotics, calcium, and vitamin D. Most importantly, it makes a great base for a snack parfait.

1. Add yogurt to a small dish or mason jar (if prepping ahead).
2. Layer with fruit and nuts in optional alternating layers.

Kitchen Tip: Seeds can be substituted for nuts. Frozen fruits work well, too!

Banana Oat Breakfast Smoothie (V, VG, DF, GF)*

Prep time: 5 minutes

Total time: 5 minutes

Yield: *1 serving*

⅓ cup rolled oats

1 frozen banana (ripe)

1 cup whole milk or plant
milk

1 tablespoon peanut or
almond butter

1 tablespoon chia seeds

1 cup fresh spinach leaves

½ teaspoon vanilla extract

½ teaspoon cinnamon

Looking for a quick smoothie from ingredients in your cupboard and fridge? Adding oats is a great way to help you sneak in more fiber and feel satisfied longer. Plant milk or whole milk work as the base.

1. Place oats in the bottom of the blender and pulse a few times until finely ground. Add in the banana, milk, nut butter, chia seeds, spinach, vanilla, and cinnamon.
2. Blend until smooth and creamy. Add water or ice to thin if desired.

---

*Vegan and dairy free if plant milk is used. Gluten free if gluten-free oats are used.

Kitchen Tip: Unsweetened soy, pea, or flax milk work well in this recipe.

Alma's Story

Alma and Diego had been married about five years and were ready to start a family. She enjoyed her job as a dental hygienist and loved to plan her future. She talked to her doctor about trying to conceive and was advised to "give it a year." Sadly, for Alma the year passed without a positive pregnancy test. She felt frustrated and followed up with her doctor. He ran lab tests and diagnosed her with PCOS. She was surprised because her periods were regular, though very heavy and painful. She had not planned for this!

This news was emotionally difficult for Alma, and she wanted to start treatments. She was prescribed medications for three cycles, which not only made her feel terrible, but she did not get pregnant. She educated herself about PCOS from podcasts and was "hearing conflicting information on what to eat." PCOS content on social media stressed her out. Finally, she talked to her brother who was into health and fitness. He talked to his nutritionist, who knew that Judy specialized in reproductive nutrition.

Alma learned about our Food for Fertility class, which was starting in just over a month. "I'm a little bit picky and don't tolerate dairy; I was worried about the foods in class," Alma recalled. But she found it was really fun, and dairy wasn't required. "When I started hearing everyone's story, I felt more comfortable. Working together with women in a hands-on environment felt empowering." Alma felt she was in the right place to focus on self-care to help her get pregnant.

She tried almost every recipe at home, and instantly they were eating more vegetables. "I love being hands on," Alma says. "It helps me remember the recipe because I made it. We prepare more vegetables, lentils, and hearty soups." Diego was also eating much healthier by consuming fewer sweets and more fruits and vegetables. But most importantly, Alma felt she could relate to all the women in class and no longer felt alone with her infertility.

After following the Food for Fertility program for a while, Alma felt she had more energy and was no longer feeling sluggish. She learned not to feel guilty if she ate a treat and felt the class provided accountability for her new habits. Classes also helped her to become more mindful. She appreciated the ability to acknowledge her hunger and fullness and learn to respect them.

One night, about a month into taking the class, Alma couldn't sleep. She decided to take a pregnancy test. A faint line appeared, but she just wasn't sure about the results. Alma took a second test, and it was positive! Alma experienced nausea pretty quickly into her pregnancy and was nervous the cooking smells in class might be too much, but she was happy to finish the class series, especially after Judy assured her it would provide a great foundation for her pregnancy. After trying to conceive for two years, she was thrilled to be a mom.

Alma and Diego wanted to share their gender reveal with friends and family both live and globally, all the way to their family in Brazil. With the help of her doctor, they were able to have Seattle's giant Ferris wheel turn pink!

Takeaways

1. A cup or less of high-fat dairy per day may be beneficial for a woman's ovulation.
2. Plant milk provides an alternative to dairy. Soy milk has the most fertility benefits. Look for unsweetened varieties that have calcium added.
3. Vitamin D is important for reproductive health, and vitamin D deficiency may be detrimental to some metabolic and endocrine functions. Supplement if your levels are low.
4. Fermented dairy such as yogurt and kefir, along with other fermented foods like sauerkraut and kimchi, benefit gut health and reproductive health.

Sample SMART Goals

1. Try a recipe with whole-fat yogurt or a plant-based yogurt this week.
2. Add a tablespoon of kimchi to an egg scramble or lunch bowl for gut health.
3. Add a tablespoon of sauerkraut to a bowl of beans and greens for a fertility-friendly meal.

Chapter 7

Animal Proteins (Beef, Pork, Lamb, Poultry, Eggs)

Test Your Knowledge

*Protein powder is needed in smoothies to get enough protein.** True/False*
*It's easy to get enough protein on a plant-forward diet.*** True/False*

I n the United States, we have a love affair with protein. It is the darling of macronutrients, unlike fats and carbs, which have both been disparaged by diet trends. No one ever says, "I'm eating low protein," although plenty of people are proud to proclaim they are eating low carb or low fat. What is going on? Our bodies need carbohydrates for energy and fat to build cell membranes and sex hormones. We need amino acids from proteins to build tissue in our body. But have we gone overboard with meat?

---

* False. Healthy smoothies can use full protein sources such as yogurt, dairy, soy or protein milks, nut butter, seeds, silken tofu, chia seeds, or ricotta cheese!

** True. Beans, lentils, soy, dairy, grains, and vegetables all contain adequate protein. Plus, many people on a plant-forward diet still consume plenty of eggs, dairy, and fish.

Protein can make up anywhere from 10 to 30 percent of a typical diet worldwide. Most reproductive-aged adults weighing between 150 and 200 pounds need about 50 to 70 grams of protein per day. But many people consume much more than they need, and most of this protein comes from animal sources. Of course, the amount of protein a person needs will depend on their size, age, activity level, and personal preference. The trouble with ingesting too much protein is that the body does not have a way to store it once all needs are met, so any excess protein will convert to fat for long-term energy storage, just like any extra carbohydrate or fat would. Too much protein can also cause a strain on your bones and kidneys over time.

Health Effects of Meat

The beneficial nutrients in meat include high amounts of protein, B vitamins, zinc, iron, choline, and selenium. The quantity of protein and minerals from a serving of meat is much higher than what is typically found in a serving of plants.

Eating meat at a meal is part of many food cultures and quantity of consumption frequently parallels a country's economic wealth. Levels of meat consumption are highest in the United States compared to other countries. However, eating large amounts may not be in one's best interest in the long run. Red meat (any mammalian muscle meat including beef, pork, lamb, veal, and goat) and processed meats (salami, bacon, and hot dogs) can contribute to chronic inflammation, which can increase risk of cardiovascular disease[1] and a higher risk of cancer.[2]

What about poultry and fish? Aside from fried chicken, which like all fried foods is inflammatory, cooked poultry does not appear to contribute to inflammation, and fatty fish appears to be anti-inflammatory. However, chicken consumption has been linked to heart disease (but not cancer).[3] Fish has not been connected to a higher risk of cancer or cardiovascular disease, so it appears to be the healthiest choice when it comes to animal-sourced protein.

Why does much of the evidence show that a diet high in animal fat and protein causes harm to our health over time? It is hard to know definitively, and there are likely many contributing factors. One factor may be that when people frequently eat meat, they may be eating fewer fiber-rich legumes and vegetables. Foods derived from animal flesh contain zero fiber, depriving the trillions of microbes that live in our gut the nutrition they are counting on. The immune system will be stressed and triggered when the gut is damaged from a weak microbiome, creating a chronic inflammatory state. This inflammatory state is the basis of most chronic diseases including diabetes, hypertension, autoimmune diseases, cardiovascular disease, cancers, dementia, and some causes of infertility.

In some Asian countries, where the consumption of meat is much lower and the consumption of vegetables and legumes is much higher, these chronic diseases are not seen nearly as often. Maybe the higher risk of these chronic diseases in the United States is due to the higher quantities of meat consumed daily, or maybe the quality of the meat is not as good. Perhaps it's due to the lack of more protective vegetables and legumes. What we do know from observational studies is that people who follow a plant-based diet see fewer of these diseases.

Diet Trends to Avoid

Diets that emphasize animal protein and severely curtail legumes and grains, such as the ketogenic (keto) diet, Whole 30, or the Paleo diet, increase foods from animal sources while missing out on foods that contain important micronutrients to support sperm and egg development. A keto diet may be one of the worst diets for fertility because it increases inflammatory animal proteins (without fiber) and eliminates almost all carbohydrates, including fruits, most vegetables, grains, and legumes—exactly the opposite of what has been shown to correlate with the highest fertility rates. This diet will likely result in nutritional deficiencies and reduce fertility potential.

Another diet pattern to avoid while trying to conceive is intermittent fasting or time-restricted eating. By restricting food intake to only an eight-hour window per day, you may be missing important nutrients for reproductive health. Fasting overnight for twelve hours is perfectly fine, but sixteen or more hours of fasting is not recommended while trying to conceive.

Health Benefits of Eggs

Eggs pack an amazing amount of nutrients in a small package. They provide protein and contain important nutrients like vitamin A, vitamin D, vitamin E, vitamin B12, selenium, and choline. One egg supplies a day's worth of the amino acid leucine, which is important for muscle recovery.

Fertility Research

Let's look again at the original study that established the first fertility diet. This survey revealed that women who ate a diet high in fruits, vegetables, and plant proteins had less ovulatory infertility than those who ate a more typical Western diet with more fast food and trans-fats.[4] Additional studies have shown that closer adherence to a plant-forward dietary pattern, emphasizing fruits, vegetables, grains, legumes, olive oil, fish, and poultry, leads to a higher chance of pregnancy during IVF treatment.[5] Similarly, a survey of a group of patients going through IVF demonstrated that adherence to a fertility-promoting diet, with an emphasis on seafood instead of other meats, plus soy, whole grains, fruits, vegetables, and dairy, led to higher pregnancy rates.[6] One study noted that consumption of red meat was correlated with a lower chance of blastocyst formation during IVF.[7]

What about in men? Higher consumption of saturated fat, which is seen in animal products, has been linked to lower sperm counts in males.[8] That same study also showed that higher consumption of polyunsaturated fats, such as omega-3 fatty acids found in plants and fish, showed better sperm morphology. Another paper compiling results from thirty-five studies found that diets higher in fish, poultry, grains, fruits, vegetables, and low-fat dairy were associated with better sperm quality.[9]

There are limited studies looking specifically at poultry and fertility. The Nurses' Health Study II, published in 2008, looked at more than 18,000 nurses and found that one extra serving of chicken or turkey daily was associated with a 50 percent higher risk of infertility due to lack of regular ovulation.[10] Plant-based proteins like beans, lentils, soy, and full-fat dairy had the opposite effect and decreased ovulatory infertility. In another study of more than one hundred men who were going through IVF cycles with their partners, the men who consumed the most poultry had a 13 percent higher fertilization rate during IVF. This contrasted with a lower fertilization rate seen in men who ate more processed meat.[11] So, poultry may be better than red meat or processed meat when it comes to your fertility, but it's not as good as fish or plant-based proteins. Women who don't ovulate regularly may want to reduce their poultry consumption.

Although there are not any direct studies correlating egg consumption and fertility, many people who follow a plant-forward, whole-food diet include eggs. Choline, a nutrient found in eggs, is important for reproduction in women. About three eggs per week will provide enough choline for optimal (human) egg development.

The table below shows our best assessment, based on the current research, regarding protein sources and their correlation with fertility.

Fertility Correlation with Different Protein Sources

Higher Fertility	Neutral	Reduced Fertility
Beans	Eggs	Processed meat
Lentils	Dairy	Red meat
Soy	Poultry	Poultry (if anovulatory)
Fish		

Shopping for Meat

We know that many people enjoy eating meat and poultry. And most individuals likely imagine their meat source having previously lived an idyllic life, wandering outside on a farm rather than being stuck inside in a very tight space. The free-range animals you may be envisioning roaming around outside exist, but it costs more to raise them this way. Most grocery stores, fast-food restaurants, and other casual restaurants offer less expensive, factory-raised, grain-fed meat, which is not as nutrient dense. The meat from a single ground beef patty, which may include meat that comes from one hundred different cows, is likely to pose a greater health risk than a single small steak.

If you currently eat red meat, seek out the highest quality you can find, specifically grass-fed or free-range livestock at your grocer or butcher shop. These animals will have higher levels of omega-3s and naturally occurring vitamins A, D, and K, and will pass those nutrients on to you. Or look for meat that comes from animals that were hunted in the wild. Eating small amounts of higher-quality meat from animals who were not subject to stressful living conditions, and without hormones or antibiotics, will provide more nutrients for your body, taste better, and pose fewer health risks.

Labeling rules for chickens make it difficult for you to know how the chicken was raised. Only chickens labeled "pasture raised" have room to roam outdoors under less stressful conditions, with each chicken allotted approximately 108 square feet. Free-range, cage-free, and organic-labeled chickens are confined to much smaller spaces, typically two feet or less, creating stressful conditions for the animals. Pasture-raised chickens are not given hormones or antibiotics. Their flesh is better for you and more sustainable, and the conditions are certainly better for the chickens. This higher-quality meat can be found at farmers markets or online. If you can't access pasture raised, your next best choice would be organic, free-range, antibiotic-free chicken.

The animal agriculture industry has made meat less healthy for us. From a health standpoint, if you're a regular carnivore, we encourage you to decrease your weekly consumption of factory-farmed meat and poultry to boost your fertility. Although it is more expensive, sustainably raised meat and poultry has more nutrient density. The added expense will be worth the benefit of improving your health. And realistically, your weekly grocery bill may be about the same if you replace some of the industrial meat with less expensive beans and lentils.

Shopping for Eggs

Like chicken labels, egg labels can be difficult to interpret. When shopping for eggs, look for "pasture raised." Pasture raised means that the hens laying the eggs are given access to a pasture for roaming. "Certified humane" is another good label to look for. It means the chickens are given a certain amount of space and low exposure to ammonia, which is important to minimize toxicity in the resulting eggs. Organic eggs have not been exposed to pesticides, hormones, or antibiotics, and the hens that lay them are cage free at a minimum. Some eggs are labeled as "vegetarian," which may seem a bit strange, since chickens normally graze on bugs and rodents outdoors, but it just means that their additional feed is limited to vegetarian sources.

Of course, costs will vary, but for the best balance between nutrition and cost, we recommend pasture-raised and/or organic eggs. Organic pasture-raised eggs are ideal when you are trying to conceive because you avoid hormones, antibiotics, and pesticides. These will be the highest-quality, most nutrient-dense eggs.

Nutritional Spotlight: Choline

Choline is important for many biological processes. It provides methyl groups that are important for many metabolic pathways. It helps support the structural integrity of cell membranes, neurotransmitter function, modulating gene expression, and early brain development. Humans cannot make enough choline naturally, so much of it needs to come from diet or supplementation. The main sources of choline in the diet are animal sources: eggs, meat, poultry, and fish. Individuals who do not eat eggs or animal products should take a choline supplement, 350 milligrams daily, to meet their nutritional needs.

Cooking Meat and Health Effects

Does the way you cook meat make a difference in health risk? Yes, it does. Dry cooking, such as grilling, roasting, or frying, leads to a nonenzymatic reaction between glucose and proteins, resulting in something called the Maillard reaction. This attractive browning of meat that most people enjoy results in the unfortunate production of advanced glycation end products (AGEs), which increase inflammation, insulin resistance, metabolic dysfunction, and oxidative stress.[12] These conditions are known to increase the risk of diabetes and cancer.[13,14] In a small study, women with PCOS who ate a diet with a higher amount of AGEs also demonstrated higher insulin resistance, testosterone levels, and oxidative stress.[15] Similarly, the effects of AGEs have been studied during IVF cycles in women with PCOS, and they have been shown to cause disruption in the ovarian microenvironment, negatively impacting egg quality.[16]

The Protein Flip and Swap

A typical diet in the United States has meat as the anchor of the lunch and dinner plate. Meals are built around the protein, with side dishes to accent the meat. Many people eat meat two or three times a day. The U.S. Department of Agriculture, which keeps track of the average meat and poultry consumption, reports an average of about one to two pounds of beef and pork per person weekly, plus more than an additional pound of chicken per person, per week.[17] This much animal protein and fat intake can cause chronic inflammation in the gut, which can stress the metabolic and reproductive systems. The high global demand for beef is also a main source of greenhouse gas emissions and deforestation of the world's rainforests.[18]

Two approaches that can encourage a reduction in the consumption of meat are a protein flip[19] and a protein swap.[20] The idea behind them is to reduce your weekly consumption of meat by 25 to 50 percent for personal health benefits (and the health of the planet)[21] without giving up your favorite foods or traditions.

The protein *flip* concept moves meat to a supporting role and builds the meal around nutrient-dense vegetables, whole grains, and legumes. This idea may be quite novel for some. With the protein flip, a typical four-ounce portion of meat may become a two-ounce portion, and complement the flavor of a meal instead of standing alone. Rather than just have two ounces of isolated meat on your plate, try sprinkling pieces of meat over a colorful salad or grain bowl. When you're at the market, instead of buying a pound of meat, try buying half a pound, and think about combining it with half a pound of beans or lentils in a dish. You can eat a portion for dinner and save the rest as a freezer meal.

The concept of the protein *swap* is to forego the animal protein altogether for a few meals during the week and replace it with a plant-based protein like beans, lentils, or tofu. This is the concept behind "meatless Mondays" and even "Veganuary" (vegan January) challenges. Sometimes meat eaters choose to try a meat analogue—a plant-based food that is meant to mimic meat. These meat analogues are processed and frequently high in fat and additives, so they aren't a great long-term solution for health, but they can be a transitional option if you want to try them as a swap. There are also more traditional veggie burgers, hot dogs, and roasts available that are not meant to mimic meat in cooking characteristics or flavor. Also a good swap option, they may use soy, seitan (wheat gluten), or jackfruit as their protein component.

Let's say you enjoy meat as the main part of your meal for lunch and dinner every day. Perhaps you'd consider replacing a meat dish with a spicy lentil curry, a black bean and roasted red pepper burrito, or a cabbage and tofu stir-fry. Sounds pretty yummy, right?

Decreasing your meat consumption does not require you to become vegetarian. A common description for someone who is mainly plant-based but continues to enjoy meals with meat is a "flexitarian." It allows for personal flexibility. You can eat a primarily plant-forward diet while continuing to incorporate smaller servings of meat a few times per week and still get the advantages of high-fiber vegetables and legumes.

Many medical conditions may be delayed or prevented by eating less protein from animals and sticking mainly, but not exclusively, to whole plant foods. And, as you've seen, reducing meat and incorporating more veggies and beans in your diet will enhance your odds of pregnancy now. Eating a pro-fertility diet during the peak of adulthood can shorten time to pregnancy and prevent or delay many long-term problems such as diabetes, hypertension, cardiovascular disease, and cancer. Visualize your older self, thanking your younger self for taking such good care of the body that you both share. If you are a regular meat eater, think about giving the protein flip or swap a try!

Adding New Protein Anchors

If you're inspired to reduce your meat intake, you may be wondering: Will you be able to get enough protein from plants? This is a frequent concern we hear, and the answer is a resounding yes![22] We've provided a couple of sample menus to show you where your protein is coming from when you aren't eating a typical Western diet of meat two or three times a day.

The first sample menu incorporates the protein flip and swap to help move from an average one to two pounds of animal protein per week to less than one pound per week. The second sample menu moves further toward fish- and plant-based proteins to optimize reproductive health. This one also adds more legumes, including soy, which has been shown to have fertility benefits.

These are not meant to represent complete meals, as they only show the major protein sources. For a complete meal illustration, see the sample Food-First Fertility menus on pages 226–230. Also, note that vegetables, grains, nuts, and seeds contribute additional protein.

Protein Flip and Swap Menu

	Sunday	Monday	Tuesday
Breakfast	Egg and tempeh bacon	Whole-fat yogurt	Egg and chicken or veggie sausage
Lunch	4 ounces black beans	3 ounces tuna	Hummus
Dinner	3 ounces salmon	3 ounces chicken	2 ounces beef, 2 ounces beans

Plant-Forward, Pro-Fertility Protein Menu

	Sunday	Monday	Tuesday
Breakfast	Egg and tempeh bacon	Whole-fat yogurt	Nut butter on whole grain toast
Lunch	4 ounces black beans	3 ounces tuna	Hummus
Dinner	3 ounces salmon	4 ounces tofu	4 ounces lentils

Nutritional Spotlight: Vitamin B12

Vitamin B12 is needed for DNA formation, cell division, red blood cell formation, nerve function, and metabolism. Generally, it comes from farmed animal sources that have been given vitamin B12 supplements. It is naturally present in bacteria in soil or water, so some farming practices may lead to some vitamin B12 development. Some cereals and plant milks have vitamin B12 added. Tempeh and nutritional yeast are two of the few true plant foods that naturally contain B12. There is a higher rate of vitamin B12 deficiency in people who are vegetarian, those with malabsorption issues, and those who take certain medications. Metformin or acid reducers can reduce absorption of vitamin B12, and the absorption of vitamin B12 also decreases generally after about age fifty. If your diet is mainly plant-based, if you are on metformin or acid reducers, or if you have a significant gastrointestinal condition affecting absorption, ask to have your vitamin B12 level checked. Cyanocobalamin, marketed as vitamin B12, is very stable and may be taken as pills, drops, or sublingually.

Culinary Spotlight: Umami

Umami is one of our five core tastes, along with salty, sweet, bitter, and sour. Whereas most people can identify the other four tastes, umami is a little vague. It is best described as savory or meaty. When individuals eliminate meat from a meal, they may notice less gustatory pleasure. They may sense something lacking. Because of this, it is a good idea to know different sources of umami to include in a dish to give it that savory taste. Mushrooms, tomatoes, and seaweed can all highlight umami. Miso and soy sauce can bring a deeper savory flavor. Fish, seafood, and Parmesan cheese also add umami punch. Finally, experiment with monosodium glutamate (MSG). Glutamate basically is what our umami receptors sense, so using MSG increases the taste of umami in foods where it is typically not present. Sprinkle in a little when cooking a vegetable dish, as you would with salt. It can substitute for some of the salt content while cooking. By increasing the umami sensation, your plant-based dish may become all the more craveable and delicious.

Garden Frittata (VG, GF)

Prep time: 15 minutes
Cook time: 20 minutes
Total time: 35 minutes

Yield: 4 servings

2 tablespoons extra-virgin
  olive oil
½ cup shallots, peeled and
  thinly sliced
1 pound thin-spear
  asparagus, tough ends
  snapped off, spears cut
  diagonally into 1-inch
  pieces
6 large eggs
¾ cup ricotta cheese (can
  substitute fresh goat
  cheese, vegan cheese, or
  soft tofu)
1 tablespoon fresh chives or
  scallions, minced
¼ teaspoon dried tarragon
¼ cup grated Parmesan or
  Gruyère cheese
Salt and pepper

There is no end to what you can add to a frittata. Any vegetables on hand will do. We made this one in the spring when the asparagus was just coming into its season. Enjoy it for breakfast, lunch, or dinner with a pile of beautiful delicate greens dressed with a light lemon vinaigrette!

1. Heat olive oil in a 9- or 10-inch oven-proof frying pan over medium heat. Add shallots and sauté, stirring occasionally, until they turn translucent, about 3 minutes.

2. Add asparagus and a pinch of salt. Cook for an additional 3 minutes.

3. In a medium bowl, whisk eggs, ricotta cheese, and a pinch of salt and pepper. Stir in chives and tarragon.

4. Pour the egg mixture into the pan and cook on medium-low heat until it is almost set, but still runny on top, about 4 to 5 minutes. While cooking, preheat the oven broiler.

5. Sprinkle grated cheese on top of the egg mixture.

6. Place the frying pan a couple of inches under the broiler until the cheese is melted and browned, and the center of the frittata is set (non-jiggly), about 5 to 8 minutes. Remove the pan from the oven with oven mitts.

7. Let cool for 5 to 10 minutes. Slide the frittata onto a serving plate. Cut into 6 pieces and serve.

Lentil Chili (V, VG, DF, GF)

Prep time: 15 minutes
Cook time: 40 minutes
Total time: 55 minutes

Yield: 6 to 8 servings

2 tablespoons extra-virgin
    olive oil
1 medium yellow onion,
    peeled and chopped
1 red bell pepper, seeded and
    chopped
1 small jalapeño pepper,
    seeded and diced
5 garlic cloves, peeled and
    minced
4 teaspoons chili powder
1 teaspoon cumin
2¼ cups (1-pound bag)
    brown lentils, rinsed
2 (15-ounce) cans or boxes
    diced tomatoes
1 bay leaf
8 cups vegetable broth
1 teaspoon of salt and a few
    grinds of fresh pepper
¼ cup chopped cilantro
    (optional)
Sriracha or other hot sauce of
    your choice (optional)

This lentil chili can be made as a protein swap without meat, or as a protein flip with half a pound of cooked meat along with the lentils. A full serving will be plant forward, protein flipped or swapped, and fertility enhancing. Lentils cook quickly and soak up the flavor of the hearty vegetables and spices. Peppers will impart different amounts of heat. Add more if you like it spicy, or leave them out altogether, and don't forget to add your favorite toppings.

1. In a large Dutch oven, add oil over medium heat. When the oil is hot, add onion and the red and jalapeño peppers, and stir frequently until the vegetables begin to brown, about 5 to 6 minutes.

2. Add garlic, chili powder, and cumin, and stir constantly until fragrant, about 1 minute.

3. Add lentils, tomatoes, bay leaf, broth, salt, and pepper. Bring to a boil, reduce heat to medium-low, and simmer partially covered for 30 minutes or until lentils are tender.

4. Uncover the pot and cook 10 minutes longer. Remove bay leaf. Ladle into bowls and top with cilantro or other toppings as desired.

Kitchen Tips:

- Leftovers will keep in the fridge for 5 days or up to 3 months in the freezer.
- The chili will thicken as it sits; add water to thin as needed.
- Consider topping with sliced jalapeño peppers, diced avocado, lime wedges, or pickled red onions.

Katie's Story

Katie has a long and complex fertility story, but it is not uncommon for women to experience this kind of arduous journey. "I've never been the skinny one, and I'm fine with that. But it's always been hard to hear that my weight might be the reason [I couldn't conceive]." She became tearful at this point in our conversation. "I thought because I wasn't losing weight and I wasn't gaining weight, everything was fine. I didn't know that nutrition could have such a strong effect. Hearing that was difficult because you don't get told that. I would have focused on that a lot earlier if I had any idea that it had anything to do with fertility."

"We were very much a meat-and-potatoes or meat-and-rice family. And I always felt tired and heavy after eating, so I started making less. I make extra vegetables instead. We used to just eat carrots, corn, and potatoes. Now, we eat spinach, green beans, brussels sprouts, cabbage, broccoli, cauliflower, and butternut squash. I made a frittata this weekend with bacon and cheese, but I added spinach. It was delicious. I never would have had spinach in my fridge before. When I go to the farmers market, I know what a lot more of the stuff is."

It was during a break from fertility treatments that Katie and her husband spontaneously conceived. "We were trying to figure out how we could afford IVF and my brain was on overload. Having a mental break really helped. I spent a lot more time on self-care. I was doing acupuncture, too. I did a lot more for myself." Now, her baby is almost one. Everything she learned in the class was incredibly helpful to have a healthy pregnancy because she had made so many changes to her diet and lifestyle, including the protein flip and swap and adding more vegetables. "I think the class totally influenced my success. It put more focus on nutrition and how important it was. It's not about how much you weigh, it's how you treat your body, it's how active you are and what you put in your body. People are different shapes and sizes for a reason. You're not overweight because you're lazy and sitting there eating cake all day. I can eat the same things as my skinny friends who have three kids, and it doesn't make a difference. I think that's the biggest thing, once I got that in my head. It doesn't matter what size you are, just make healthy decisions. You're either going to stay the size you are, or you're not. It doesn't matter. I actually lost twenty pounds, but it wasn't easy. I worked my butt off! I think working out and focusing on what I was eating really helped." The new habits from the class stuck. She maintained that her whole-food, plant-forward flexitarian diet and regular exercise routine ultimately led to her success. As she prepares for baby number two, she knows exactly what she needs to do.

Takeaways

1. Red meat is linked to lower fertility in women and men.
2. Legumes, fish, and eggs are the proteins associated with the highest fertility.
3. When a diet is predominately plant-based, occasional consumption of red meat causes less inflammation than when it is consumed regularly.
4. Three pasture-raised eggs per week provide enough choline to support human egg development.

Sample SMART Goals

1. Try the protein flip. Make meat the condiment in a recipe rather than the main attraction.
2. Try the protein swap. Swap a beef burger for a veggie burger loaded with your favorite veggie toppings. See if you feel equally satisfied.
3. Try going meat-free for one or two meals a week. Make a plan for a delicious plant-based meal incorporating beans, mushrooms, and tomatoes for umami.
4. Seek out grass-fed or free-range livestock. They have higher nutrient quality.
5. Seek out pasture-raised, free-range, antibiotic-free, organic eggs, and poultry for the highest nutrient quality.
6. Add greens and other vegetables for added fiber when you are eating animal protein.

Chapter 8

Go Fish!

Test Your Knowledge

Fish is too high in mercury for me to safely eat. True/False

*Vegetarians can get omega-3 fatty acids from plant foods.*** True/False

Fish is the least consumed animal protein but may be the most benefi-cial. According to the National Oceanic and Atmospheric Administra-tion (NOAA), average per capita fish and shellfish consumption in the United States is only nineteen pounds per person annually.[1] That's about one and a half servings per person per week. Fish*** is low in saturated fat, is high in protein, and is an excellent source of many nutrients.

---

* False. There are many fish that are low in mercury. Enjoy two to three servings of fish a week if you choose smaller, low-mercury fish such as salmon, trout, shellfish, and sardines, and you will reap the great taste and the best omega-3 benefits.

** True. Alpha-linolenic acid (ALA) is a plant-based omega-3 that is in walnuts, chia seeds, and flaxseeds, as well as beans and canola oil. However, ALA has less than 10 percent of the omega-3 benefits that fish sources of omega-3 have.

*** When we refer to fish, we typically mean both fish and shellfish. When we say fatty fish, that spe-cifically refers to the oily fish species that contain more of the omega-3 fatty acids like salmon, mackerel, sardines, and anchovies, among others.

We want to dispel some of the myths about fish and show you how easy, delicious, and nutritious it can be in a plant-forward diet. As with most things, you can benefit from being a wise consumer of fish and shellfish. We will teach you how to enjoy fish safely and sustainably and give you some easy recipes so you can welcome more fish into your diet.

Health Benefits

Fish and shellfish are good sources of protein, omega-3 fatty acids, selenium, iron, zinc, magnesium, choline, iodine, vitamins B6 and B12, niacin, and vitamin D. Fatty fish with higher omega-3 content can be even more beneficial for cardiovascular health and to lower blood pressure.[2] A large analysis showed that eating only one to two servings of fatty fish per week reduced the risk of dying from heart disease by 36 percent.[3] Eating fish may also be helpful for brain health and reducing the risk of dementia, as well as decreasing the risk of some autoimmune diseases.

Fertility Benefits

Does eating fish make you more fertile? Likely so. Fish is part of a nutritious diet to support preconception health. There are quite a few studies that have looked at fish consumption and fertility outcomes. One study followed about five hundred couples from Texas and Michigan participating in the Longitudinal Investigation of Fertility and the Environment study and had them record the number of seafood servings eaten in a cycle, along with sexual frequency, and time to pregnancy.[4] Women and men who ate eight or more servings of seafood per month had a shorter time to pregnancy than the couples who ate seafood one or fewer times per month. The couples who ate fish eight or more times per month also had 22 percent higher rates of sexual intercourse. So, couples who ate the most seafood had more sex and a shorter time to pregnancy. Go fish!

Another study surveyed a group of Spanish graduate students and found that those who followed a Western-style diet had more difficulty conceiving than those who ate a Mediterranean diet consisting of fruits and vegetables, grains, and fish.[5] A third study looked at a group of 155 men. They were asked to complete a food-frequency questionnaire and then provided semen samples. Fish intake, notably more than 2.4 servings per week, was related to higher sperm count and a higher percentage of normal morphology (shape of sperm). Higher consumption of processed meat was associated with lower morphology scores.[6] In a different study, people who consumed more fish had better blastocyst formation and embryo quality observed in an IVF lab.[7]

The EARTH study looked at different sources of animal proteins to see how they affected fertility in more than three hundred women undergoing ART (assisted reproductive technology, such as IVF) treatment. The average consumption of meat or fish was about one serving per day. Poultry was eaten most frequently, followed by fish, processed meat, and then red meat. Only the intake of fish was positively correlated with live birth. When researchers estimated fish replacing any other meat for two of the participants' meals per week, the increase in projected live birth was 50 percent.[8] Because fish contain a high amount of free fatty acids, this micronutrient may be looked at as a surrogate marker for fish consumption. Free fatty acids were measured in one hundred women in the EARTH study on days three and nine of an IVF cycle. Women who had higher levels of omega-3 fatty acids had about an 8 percent higher rate of pregnancy and live birth.[9,10]

Interestingly, two more observational studies looking at large cohorts of women trying to conceive naturally, one in Denmark and one in North America, showed no difference in pregnancy rates with different levels of fish consumption while trying to conceive for up to a year[11]—meaning that, in these two studies, the effect of seafood appeared neutral overall. For those who do not or cannot eat fish, this study could be considered reassuring that they are not at a disadvantage.

The North American cohort looked at how the seafood was cooked as well. They noted lower fertility rates in consumers of fried shellfish compared to nonfried shellfish. They concluded that deep frying fish could counterbalance any positive or neutral health effects—a bit of a bummer for those who enjoy their fish and chips!

Mercury in Fish

Mercury and other contaminants in fish can be harmful at high levels, affecting the central and peripheral nervous system.[12] Mercury does not naturally leave your body, and public health messages warn people to reduce mercury exposure, especially during pregnancy. This leads many people to limit all fish consumption, rather than limiting just those with the highest levels of mercury. However, eliminating all fish consumption in pregnancy means missing out on some important nutrients, since omega-3 fatty acids improve fetal brain development.

Individuals need to know which fish are healthful and safe to eat, and which may pose more risk.[13] Mercury accumulates in larger predatory fish such as king mackerel, bigeye tuna, shark, swordfish, orange roughy, tilefish, and marlin. Most smaller fish like sardines and anchovies, as well as shellfish, salmon, and trout, have low mercury levels and are safe to eat. The American College of Obstetrics and Gynecology recommends limiting consumption of fish with the highest mercury levels to one serving or less per week for women trying to conceive and those who are pregnant.[14] Low-mercury fish may be consumed two or three times per week. It is quite easy to stay well within safe levels and consume eight to twelve ounces of fish per week to get the fertility benefits.[15,16] Overall, consuming low-mercury fish while trying to conceive is not only safe but recommended.[17]

Concerns About Sustainability and Pollutants in Fish

Mercury isn't the only concern many have when it comes to fish and shellfish. Many species are over fished, which is detrimental to our oceans and the environment. Also, much of our current fish supply is less healthy not due to mercury, but due to pollution of our waterways. Lakes and rivers can be polluted, and oceans are becoming acidified. Pollutants get into our fish and, from there, into us.

One way to learn more about fish, shop sustainably, and avoid contaminants is to refer to the Monterey Bay Aquarium's Seafood Watch website at seafoodwatch.org. They regularly update their pocket guide, which you can use while shopping, or ask your grocer about it when at your local market.[18] You can also look for the Marine Stewardship Council (MSC) stamp for sustainability.

Shopping for Fish

Fish have seasons, just like produce. It is best to buy fish when it is in season or buy it when it has been frozen right after it is caught.

Salmon is a favorite for many and is usually fresh in summer. Sockeye and coho are the species that are frequently eaten as an everyday fillet. Pink salmon and keta may be sold in cans or jars and added to chowder. Salmon fillets have pin bones that should be removed from your fillet before cooking. Otherwise, look for small bones while eating. Tail fillets have no bones to worry about.

More sustainable fishing practices have allowed wild salmon to exist but not flourish as it once did. Chinook, or king salmon, is the main food source for orca whales in the Pacific Northwest. Unfortunately, climate, pollution, dams, and fishing practices have led to a major decline in the king salmon population and thus a critical decline in the population of orcas. Many people choose to avoid purchasing or eating king salmon to leave the remaining supply for the orca population. We also recommend you avoid farm-raised salmon in net pens if you can. They can spread disease, and if they escape, they compete with wild salmon.

White fish such as cod, halibut, flounder, haddock, and tilapia are mild in flavor and low in fat. Trout can be wild or farmed: wild rainbow trout are from the Pacific Northwest, and much of the available rainbow trout is sustainably farmed in Idaho and available year-round. Rainbow trout lends itself well to cooking in a cast iron skillet, leading to a crispy skin and delicately cooked flesh. Another fish to try is wild black cod from Alaska. Although you can buy farmed black cod, wild is best—it's full of fat and omega-3s. Black cod is delicious roasted with a miso and mirin marinade.

Shrimp is now sustainably caught in the Pacific Ocean. Depending on the type and where you live, you may get some shrimp freshly caught, but shrimp is always available year-round in the freezer. Frozen shrimp thaw very quickly and can be used to make a high-protein meal on a weeknight. Prawns require a little effort to enjoy because they need to be peeled and sometimes deveined before eating. Once you know how, it can be quite fun and worth it!

Little fish include sardines, anchovies, squid, mackerel, and herring. They are full of omega-3s, vitamin D, and protein and have the lowest levels of mercury and toxins since they eat mostly plankton. Sardine fisheries are sustainable, and sardines are available year-round in tins, although you may sometimes be lucky and find them in glass jars, which allows you to decrease your exposure to BPA. Other fish may also be found in glass jars as well, including salmon, tuna, and anchovies. To prepare sardines, we split them in half and pull the spine out. Then we add them to a salad or an open-face sandwich with some lovely greens for a delicious lunch. Anchovies are saltier than sardines or mackerel and can add some great umami to a sauce or dressing. We chop them up and add them to salad dressings and tomato-based sauces.

Cooking Fish

The key to enjoying fish is to learn to cook fish well. It's not hard once you know how. Many people don't like fish because they've only had it overcooked, when it becomes dreadfully dry and tasteless. To tell if your fillet is done (and not overdone), check the flake—the term used to describe the layers of the fish starting to separate. If it flakes, it means that the fish is done, but still moist and juicy.

The safety risks from cooked fish are minimal. Eating raw fish such as sushi poses a small risk as it can harbor bacteria or parasites. Once pregnant, you should avoid eating raw fish.

Culinary Spotlight: Meal Planning

Time and again, we hear from our participants that weekly meal planning and having go-to recipes are the keys to their success in eating a fertility-promoting diet. It is also part of becoming a competent eater. If you take the time to plan your meals and shop once on the weekend and a second time midweek, you will have the food you need readily available to support your reproductive health. You will be less tempted to eat out or heat up a processed meal from the freezer. Pick enough recipes for a few days' worth of meals and plan your next shopping trip.

Sunday is our big day for meal planning, shopping, prepping, and cooking. Real food takes time, and Sunday works best for us. You can pick a different day, but we suggest you commit to a routine with one day focused on food. If you plan well on Sunday, you'll have plenty of good food to carry you through at least half the week.

Nutritional Spotlight: Omega-3s

Omega-3s are important for our neurological growth and development; they have great health benefits and reduce risk of inflammation, diabetes, depression, attention-deficit hyperactivity disorder (ADHD), and dementia. Two particularly beneficial omega-3s, docosahexaenoic acid (DHA) and eicosapentaenoic acid (EPA) are not produced by our body, so we must obtain them from food. EPA is known to reduce triglycerides, reduce risk of cardiovascular disease, reduce inflammation, and lift mood. DHA is important for brain health and for brain and eye development in the second and third trimester of pregnancy.[19] Thankfully, both of these fantastic nutrients are naturally occurring in seafood and algae.

To get enough omega-3 fatty acids in your diet, it is recommended that you consume a fatty fish such as salmon twice per week, or a less fatty white fish such as cod or trout three times per week. A three-ounce serving of salmon contains anywhere from 1,000 to 1,900 milligrams of omega-3s. Sole and pollack contain about 480 milligrams per serving and canned tuna contains about 170 to 240 milligrams per serving.

For those who do not eat fish, ALA (alpha-linolenic acid) is a plant-based omega-3 found in flaxseeds, walnuts, and some vegetable oils. ALA is a precursor to EPA and DHA—but less than 10 percent of it is actually converted to DHA and EPA, which isn't much. Also, ALA does not offer the same brain, eye, and anti-inflammatory benefits as DHA and EPA. So, although we know that supplements do not offer the same benefits of food sources, you may want to consider taking a supplement with DHA and EPA if you don't eat fish. Look for a supplement with a United States Pharmacopeia (USP)–verified fish, krill, or algal oil and aim to take at least 300 milligrams of EPA and 300 milligrams of DHA daily in your omega-3 supplement.

Foods High in Omega-3 Fatty Acids

Food	DHA, mg per serving	EPA, mg per serving	ALA, mg per serving
Salmon, wild 3 ounces	1,220	350	0
Sardines 3 ounces	740	450	0
Mackerel 3 ounces	590	430	0
Trout, wild 3 ounces	440	400	0
Anchovies 1 ounce	258	152	0

Food	DHA, mg per serving	EPA, mg per serving	ALA, mg per serving
Cod, wild 3 ounces	100	40	0
Walnuts 1 ounce	0	0	7,600
Chia seeds 1 ounce	0	0	5,060
Flaxseed, whole 1 tablespoon	0	0	2,350

Source: National Institutes of Health (nih.gov) and U.S. Department of Agriculture, Agricultural Research Service, FoodData Central (usda.gov) 2019

Sheet Pan Salmon and Broccoli (GF, DF)

Prep time: 10 minutes
Cook time: 20 minutes
Total time: 30 minutes

Yield: 4 to 6 servings

2 tablespoons toasted sesame
    oil
1 tablespoon tamari
1 tablespoon unseasoned rice
    vinegar
½ tablespoon grated fresh
    ginger
1 medium garlic clove,
    peeled and minced
1 pound broccoli, trimmed
    and cut into 1½-inch
    pieces; cut thicker stems
    into ½-inch pieces
1 medium red onion, cut
    into 8 wedges
1–2 tablespoons extra-virgin
    olive oil
Salt
1 pound salmon filet
Lemon or lime wedges, for
    serving
1 tablespoon black sesame
    seeds

Wild salmon is delicious and a great source of omega-3 fatty acids. We typically use sockeye, but you can also use coho. Leftovers can be used the next day, warm or cold, on a salad or in a bowl. If you don't want leftovers, stick with a half-pound for two people. Leftover fresh ginger root can be stored in the freezer and pulled out when needed. Black sesame seeds have higher nutrient content than white seeds and include calcium, magnesium, iron, copper, and manganese. This sheet pan dinner pairs nicely with black or brown rice.

1. Heat the oven to 400°F. To make the glaze, whisk 2 tablespoons sesame oil with the tamari, vinegar, ginger, and garlic in a small bowl until smooth. Set the glaze aside.

2. Spread broccoli and red onion wedges on a sheet pan lined with aluminum foil. Drizzle with 1–2 tablespoons olive oil. Sprinkle with salt and roast until broccoli is bright green, about 7 to 10 minutes.

3. While the broccoli and red onions roast, place the salmon fillet on a plate and pat dry with paper towels. Remove any pin bones. Brush with olive oil and sprinkle with salt.

4. When the broccoli and red onions are ready, move them to the edges of the sheet pan, making room in the center of

the pan for the salmon. Place the fillet on the pan and brush with the glaze.

5. Return the pan to the oven and roast until the salmon is cooked through but slightly rare in the center, about 10 to 15 minutes. Depending on the thickness of the fillet, cook times will vary. Check at 8 minutes. It should start to flake apart and look less transparent when done.

6. When ready to plate, option to serve over a portion of rice or another grain. Serve a piece of salmon the size of a deck of cards (approximately 3 ounces). Add broccoli and red onion wedges. Option to squeeze some lemon or lime over the dish and salt to taste. Scatter the black sesame seeds over the salmon.

Tuna White Bean Salad (GF)

Prep time: 10 minutes

Total time: 10 minutes

Yield: 2 main servings or 4 side servings

3 tablespoons lemon juice

Pinch of salt

¼ teaspoon black pepper, freshly ground

1½ cups cannellini (white kidney) beans, rinsed

2 (3-ounce) packets chunk light tuna, drained and broken apart with a fork

¼ cup red onion, peeled and chopped

3 tablespoons fresh basil, chopped

Fresh greens (optional)

Here's another easy fish recipe that includes tuna and white beans and makes for a perfect lunch. It is safe and beneficial to eat tuna in limited quantities while trying to conceive. We like using the three-ounce packs of low-mercury tuna, but you could also use a six-ounce can of tuna. Avoid albacore tuna, which can have three times as much mercury as skipjack or light tuna.

1. Whisk lemon juice, salt, and pepper together in a medium bowl. Add beans, tuna, onion, and basil. Mix to coat well.
2. Serve alone or on a bed of greens.

Kitchen Tip: You can also include diced cucumbers, tomatoes, capers, sun-dried tomatoes, or any seasonal chopped vegetables.

Ryane's story

Ryane learned about our Food for Fertility program from a naturopathic physician she worked with once she decided to try to conceive. "I got my IUD out and started to think about pregnancy," she said. "I was thirty-one and he was forty-one, so it felt like the right time."

She was glad she received the advice to pursue nutrition therapy, take the class, and learn more about fertility. "The class changed my outlook about food. I feel more mindful about everything I eat. It doesn't feel like a diet at all." Before the class, Ryane thought the nutrition advice would be all black or white but was happy to find out that the plan wasn't so restrictive. "I can eat well without following a strict diet or counting calories."

Ryane enjoyed preparing the recipes at home. "We love the sheet pan dinners. I usually put tartar sauce on fish, but when we tried the salmon sheet pan dinner, we both loved it!" She found that when she implemented changes slowly, it was much easier. "The weekly goals were helpful," she recalled. "I am competitive—I try do my best to accomplish the goals I set for myself. Meal prep makes it easier. It helped me work through obstacles more than I could before. I am better at taking accountability and knowing the right steps forward. It is a good feeling; I have more control over my life and body now."

For Ryane, the psychological transformation from leaning into a fertility-promoting diet was just as significant as the physical one. "I feel like a stronger, more confident woman," she said. "I love showing my food at work; I have a lot of pride in how I am taking care of myself. My colleagues are so interested in what I bring [for lunch] and ask for the recipes!"

Ultimately, Ryane needed a small surgery to improve her uterine cavity before starting fertility treatments. She went on to successfully conceive after three months of medication to help with ovulation.

Takeaways

1. Most studies show that fish consumption enhances fertility.
2. Fish are the highest animal source of omega-3 fatty acids. Eating two to three 3-ounce servings of low-mercury fish while trying to conceive is safe and recommended.
3. Omega-3 fatty acids are key nutrient powerhouses for their anti-inflammatory properties and support neurological and brain health. EPA and DHA, which provide these benefits, come from seafood and algae.

Sample SMART Goals

1. Experiment with cooking fish at home. Aim to purchase sustainably raised and caught seafood from natural waters or sustainable shellfish farms.
2. Incorporate sardines or anchovies into a salad or bowl.
3. If you don't eat fish: Consider taking a USP-verified supplement with 300 mg of DHA and 300 mg of EPA daily.

Chapter 9

Fertility-Friendly Fats

Test Your Knowledge

Eating nuts will make me fat. True/False

*Low-fat and no-fat foods are better for me.*** True/False

Y ou have probably heard conflicting advice about which fats are healthy and how much you should consume: *Should I be eating more coconut oil or olive oil? How do I avoid saturated fat?* With all the information (and misinformation) out there, the question remains: What role does fat play in our fertility?

Fat comes from animal sources such as fish, seafood, meat, poultry, eggs, cheese, milk, and butter. Plant sources of fat include nuts, seeds, avocados, olives, soybeans, and oils. As we saw in the last chapter, the fatty acids contained in some fish are some of the healthiest and play an important role in a

---

* False. Nuts provide your body with primarily monounsaturated fats, protein, fiber, and many micronutrients. In fact, one ounce of nuts provides you with 56 percent of your fertility-boosting selenium needs along with other important trace minerals essential for fertility. We recommend an ounce of nuts a day because they are so nutrient dense and satisfying. Research actually supports that people who eat almonds regularly lose more weight than their non-almond-consuming peers!

** False. Many products marketed as "no fat" or "low fat" often have the same calories but more carbohydrates. Eating full fat actually allows you to feel fuller and more satisfied.

Food-First Fertility Plan. Fat is known for providing energy, richness, and a smooth texture. It helps to balance flavor profiles in a dish. How much of your food intake should come from fat? That is debatable, but, for most people, between 20 and 35 percent of your total intake is appropriate.

There are four kinds of fats: saturated, monounsaturated, polyunsaturated, and trans fats. Saturated fats are solid at room temperature—think butter, the fat in a piece of bacon, or coconut oil. Some saturated fats, especially those found in meat and cheese, may have negative health effects such as promotion of atherosclerosis and inflammation (even though some cheeses may also have some positive benefits for gut health due to the live cultures). Coconut oil contains about 80 to 90 percent saturated fat, which is why it is solid at room temperature. Lauric acid in coconut oil has antimicrobial and antifungal properties, making it useful for purposes other than cooking. It may be included in toothpaste for oral health and to reduce cavities and inflammation.

Unsaturated fats can either be monounsaturated or polyunsaturated fatty acids (also referred to as MUFA or PUFA), depending on whether they have one or two or more double bonds in their chemical structure. Monounsaturated fatty acids (omega-9s) are mainly found in olives, olive oil, avocados, avocado oil, peanuts, almonds, and cashews. Having these foods in your diet results in increased levels of HDL ("good") cholesterol and lower LDL ("bad") cholesterol. MUFAs are considered nonessential fatty acids, meaning our bodies can make them, though we can also get them from food.

Polunsaturated fatty acids (omega-3 and omega-6 fatty acids) are essential fatty acids, meaning our body does not make them and you can only get them from food or supplements. In chapter eight, we spoke in detail about the three types of omega-3 fatty acids: DHA and EPA, present in seafood and algae, and ALA, found in flaxseeds, chia seeds, and walnuts. Omega-6 fatty acids help to stabilize cell membranes. They are found in eggs, nuts, and seeds. But they are also found in higher concentrations in refined vegetable cooking oils and in ultra-processed foods, which can be harmful in high amounts.

The last type of fat, trans fats, can be artificial or natural. Artificial trans fats can be created by chemically altering vegetable oil to make it solid at room temperature. Artificial trans fats were banned from our food supply in 2018 due to their associated risk of high cholesterol and heart disease.[1,2] Naturally occurring trans fats, present in meat and dairy, do not appear to pose the same health risks.

Omega-6 to Omega-3

People eating a Western-style diet typically ingest a much higher ratio of omega-6 to omega-3 fatty acids than the 4:1 ratio that's recommended—typically greater than 16:1. This is very inflammatory and deleterious to health.

Why is that ratio so high? Because many commercially available foods (hint: restaurant foods, fast food, fried foods) and less expensive foods (snack foods) are processed using commercial-grade vegetable oils (mainly from soybean oil), which have a higher concentration of omega-6 fatty acids. Given this, the key to reducing your omega-6 to omega-3 ratio is to reduce your exposure to oils with higher amounts of omega-6 (e.g., by eating out less often or by consuming enough omega-3 fatty acids such as fatty fish).

Health Benefits

We need fat in our diets to absorb and transport our fat-soluble vitamins A, D, E, and K, and to supply essential fatty acids required for health. Fatty acids are needed for production of cholesterol, sex hormones, and cell membranes. A storage form that can be converted to energy, fat also provides the padding between our organs for protection. Fat slows gastric emptying and, when eaten with carbohydrates, can delay absorption of glucose.

Multiple studies have shown that plant-based fats are healthier than animal-based fats, and including healthful plant-based fats in your diet can reduce your risk of cardiovascular disease.[3] Two large cohorts have demonstrated that higher consumers of plant-based fats showed a lower mortality rate compared to those who had higher consumption of animal-based fats.[4,5] Higher consumption of animal fats has also been shown to increase the risk of developing type 2 diabetes.[6,7]

Many of the plant foods that contain natural fat, such as nuts and avocados, bring other beneficial nutrients along with them. Olives are mainly composed of omega-9 fatty acids and have a high amount of vitamin E and strong antioxidant properties. Adding creaminess to dishes, avocados are high in omega-9 fatty acids, fiber, potassium, magnesium, and B6.

Fertility Benefits

Fat is absolutely necessary for health and fertility. It is needed to produce all your reproductive hormones like estrogen, progesterone, and testosterone. As part of the EARTH study, free fatty acids were measured in one hundred women on days three and nine of an IVF cycle. Women who had higher levels of omega-3 fatty acids had about an 8 percent higher rate of pregnancy and live birth.[8,9] Too little fat in your diet can contribute to infertility, as it can cause irregular or absent ovulation if your body doesn't have enough fat to produce reproductive hormones such as estrogen. Too much fat in your diet can impair fertility through toxicity in the ovary.[10]

There have not been any human studies specifically looking at egg quality and omega-3 levels, but in a study of aging mice, omega-3 fatty acids improved egg quality and prolonged female reproductive lifespan.[11]

Nuts

Most nuts are classified as fruits, except for peanuts, which are legumes. Nuts are an outstanding source of fat, fiber, protein, vitamins, and minerals. Common varieties of nuts include walnuts, almonds, pecans, cashews, macadamia, hazelnuts, pistachios, pine nuts, and Brazil nuts. Nuts and seeds contain monounsaturated and polyunsaturated fatty acids (MUFAs and PUFAs). Because they come from plants, they also contain phytonutrients and fiber. Nuts have been shown to lower the risk of mortality from certain diseases and benefit heart and brain health.

Many nuts and seeds contain antioxidant phytochemicals like vitamin E, ellagic acid, polyphenols, and carotenoids to protect against free radical damage. They contain high concentrations of B vitamins as well as vitamin E, which works as an antioxidant and hormone. Nuts also contain minerals like manganese, magnesium, potassium, phosphorus, calcium, iron, copper, zinc, and selenium, which all provide unique health benefits: iron is necessary for red blood cell production. Copper also helps with red blood cell production, as well as helping maintain nerve, bone, and immune health. Magnesium and phosphorus are important for bone metabolism. Manganese helps with hormone production. Zinc helps regulate growth and development, DNA synthesis, and digestion. Selenium works with antioxidant enzymes and is beneficial for sperm health.

Nutritional Spotlight: Selenium

Selenium is an essential trace mineral that is an important antioxidant for fertility. Diets higher in selenium have been found to improve sperm quality,[12] and diets that are low in selenium are associated with delayed time to pregnancy.[13] Selenium is a key nutrient in the formation of glutathione peroxidase enzyme (GPx), which plays a role in the body's detoxification processes and helps protect against oxidative stress.[14] Scientists believe that the GPx enzyme may play an important role in the development of gametes and fertilization. Although there are few studies on selenium and female fertility, studies so far appear promising.[15]

Selenium is also essential for thyroid function, which also supports fertility. Selenium works with iodine to maintain consistent thyroid function.[16] You can find excellent sources of selenium in both plants and fish. The Dietary Reference Intake (DRI) for adult women is 55 micrograms per day. Just one Brazil nut meets your daily needs!

Foods High in Selenium

	Serving size	Selenium
Brazil nuts	1 ounce	544 mcg
Tuna	3 ounces	64 mcg
Sardines	3 ounces	45 mcg
Salmon	3 ounces	40 mcg
Egg	1 egg	15 mcg

Source: U.S. Department of Agriculture, Agricultural Research Service, FoodData Central (usda.gov) 2019

Seeds

Seeds are multipurpose nutritional powerhouses, too. The seeds with the highest amount of omega-3 fatty acids include flax, hemp, and chia. Flax, chia, and sesame seeds contain lignans, which are a main source of phytoestrogens. Although there may be health benefits from lignans, they have not been well studied. Other seeds, including sesame, poppy, and Nigella, contain omega-3, omega-6, and omega-9 fatty acids and saturated fats. Seeds may benefit hormone balance, immunity, and brain health.

Cooking with Fats

Most cooking oils typically contain some combination of unsaturated and saturated fats. The oils with the highest ratio of omega-3 to omega-6 fatty acids include olive, avocado, flax, and hemp. For most of our daily cooking, we prefer olive oil or neutral-flavored oils like avocado or canola oil. The oils with the highest ratio of omega-6 include vegetable, corn, safflower, and sunflower. These are the oils we try to avoid.

Extra-virgin olive oil, or EVOO, comes from the first cold press of olives. When an oil says it is cold pressed, unrefined, or extra virgin, it means it has been less processed and retains more micronutrients, but it is also more expensive. Oils from vegetables and seeds frequently go through more chemical processing and are extracted from their source through a heated mechanical or chemical process. They are less expensive than the cold-pressed, unrefined oils, but they have the disadvantage of a higher concentration of omega-6 fatty acids. The more refined or chemically processed the oils are, the more heat tolerability they have.

You can buy EVOO from different regions such as Spain, Italy, Greece, or California. Each area will have different dominant varietals of olives, which gives the oil its distinct, floral taste. Although it has great oxidative stability, because of its expense and taste profile, it is best to use EVOO at lower temperatures when cooking, or to marinate, flavor, or finish a dish. Olive oil that comes from a later press will have a higher smoke point and will cost less than EVOO. This olive oil is perfect for cooking, roasting, or grilling. All olive oil has a high concentration of monounsaturated omega-9 fatty acids (MUFA) and is a staple in the Mediterranean diet. It also contains omega-6 fatty acids, saturated fat, and omega-3 fatty acids. How much olive oil contributes to health is debatable, but as part of a plant-forward, whole-food diet, it has been shown to lead to a lower risk of heart attack and stroke.

Avocado oil also has a high concentration of omega-9 fatty acids and also contains some omega-6 and omega-3 fatty acids. Extra-virgin, or unrefined, avocado oil has one of the highest smoke points and is one of our favorites for low-heat or high-heat cooking when we want a neutral flavor. Extra-virgin avocado oil has a higher smoke point and is great for high-temperature cooking such as stir-frying or roasting. When oil starts smoking, it can break down, become acrid, and release free radicals, which are damaging to our cells.

Canola oil is from the rapeseed plant, is commonly used by home cooks, and has a medium-high smoke point. It has a mix of mainly monounsaturated fatty acids, omega-6 and omega-3 fatty acids, and saturated fat. Its ratio of omega-6 to omega-3 is 2:1, which is better than most other oils, but canola oil has typically gone through chemical processing. It has been studied as part of the healthy, plant-forward Nordic diet where it has shown some ability to decrease blood pressure.

Vegetable oil is typically a blend of soybean and other oils. This is the most common oil in fast-food frying due to its low cost, but it has a high concentration of the more inflammatory omega-6 fatty acids.

Refined peanut oil is made up of MUFA and has high levels of omega-6s and saturated fat. It is not the healthiest choice due to the high omega-6 levels, but it imparts a nutty flavor, has a higher smoke point, and is occasionally used for frying or stir-frying.

Grapeseed oil is another neutral oil with a high smoke point, but it also has a higher concentration of omega-6 fatty acids.

Unrefined coconut oil has a lower smoke point and should be reserved for baking or sautéing and will impart a signature flavor. Because of its high saturated fat content, coconut oil is best used infrequently.

Naturally Fatty Foods

A delicious stone fruit, olives can be added to salads or in cooked dishes. Green olives are less ripe versions of black olives and have a slightly different flavor. As olives ripen, their color darkens. Olives with pits are typically higher quality than those that have had their pits removed. Add them to salads and other dishes to impart a savory, salty flavor. They are great as a stand-alone snack or can be blended with a few other ingredients to make a yummy dip.

Avocados are another delicious fruit that can be enjoyed a number of ways. Alone with a squeeze of lemon and salt, smashed on whole grain toast with a shake of sesame seeds, or smashed with garlic, lime, tomatoes, and salt as guacamole, they are a savory, nutritious snack or addition to a meal. Avocados can ripen on the counter or be stored in the refrigerator to slow ripening. Most of the avocados in the United States come from Mexico. When available, try to support fair trade farming, and look for avocados grown in California during their peak season in the spring and summer.

Olive Extravaganza! Tapenade

Tapenade is a dish originating from the Provencal region of France and is tradi-tionally a spread of black olives, anchovies, and capers puréed with olive oil. It's very easy to prepare in a small food processor. Combine one cup of kalamata olives (or 1/2 black and 1/2 green olives), an anchovy fillet (or a teaspoon of an-chovy paste), a clove of peeled garlic, a teaspoon of capers, a glug of olive oil, and a few tablespoons of lemon juice for an amazing spread, delicious on whole grain crackers or vegetables.

Eating Nuts

Nuts may be eaten raw, blended, or toasted. They should be kept cool for a longer shelf life and may be stored in your refrigerator. Toast nuts on low heat, around 300°F, for about five to ten minutes, and move them around your baking sheet halfway through, or toast a handful until they become fragrant on the stovetop. Keep your eye on them and your nose on alert, so you don't overdo it. Enjoy a handful of toasted nuts as a snack with some fruit, or toss on a salad to give it crunch and depth.

Nuts can be blended into tasty butters that can be creamy and delicious additions for bowls, smoothies, sauces, or spreads for whole grain bread. Many people enjoy nut butters, including almond, cashew, and macadamia. Many varieties are available in grocery stores. Some let you grind your own peanut butter right there in the store! Peanut butter is frequently mentioned as a nut butter, although peanuts are technically a legume.

Eating Seeds

Seeds can be toasted and added to yogurt bowls or sprinkled on salads. They can be made into grain-free or whole grain crackers and eaten with a hearty soup or salad. Seeds commonly used to make crackers include pumpkin, sesame, black sesame, and sunflower. Adding fennel, coriander, or caraway seeds, and herbs like rosemary or sage, will make them even more unique. If you are going to make a whole grain cracker, try adding short grain brown rice or millet.

Seeds, like nuts, should be kept cool and may be stored in the refrigerator. Sunflower seeds, hemp seeds, flaxseeds, and chia seeds can easily be added to salads, dressings, or smoothies. They are an easy source of omega-3 and omega-6 fatty acids, providing anti-inflammatory benefits. Nutrients from flaxseeds are best absorbed when ground rather than whole.

In addition to crackers, you can give seeds a little more heft as a snack by making energy bars. These homemade bars will be full of protein and have better ingredients with fewer preservatives than store-bought bars (which can be deceptively unhealthy). These bars require no cooking, other than the initial toasting of the seeds or nuts. Simply combine toasted seeds, coconut, vanilla, and salt. Add some maple syrup or brown rice syrup for a hint of sweetness. Top with chopped dried raspberries, and your friends will be jealous!

Homemade granola is another delicious way to combine nuts and seeds for a snack. Granola is great on top of yogurt or grain cereals, or with fruit or sliced veggies in the mid-morning or afternoon. Read labels if you buy granola from a store, as it may contain high amounts of sugar and fat. The best thing is to make your own at home where you control the ingredients. Base granola recipes typically have rolled oats, unsweetened coconut, almonds or other nuts, sunflower seeds, sesame seeds, pumpkin seeds, coconut oil, brown rice syrup, vanilla, and cinnamon. From that base, dial up whichever flavors you prefer: vanilla almond, pumpkin spice, or cacao nibs are all easy options to add.

Chia pudding is another easy snack to make at home. Combine chia seeds with a nut milk and let the mixture sit for a few hours or overnight. You can then add fresh fruit as a topping.

Culinary Spotlight: Spices

Spices are a key component of your culinary repertoire that can really elevate your cooking. Combinations of spices will give distinct flavor profiles to your dishes and provide added health benefits from polyphenols.[17,18] Many spices have active antioxidant properties like the curcumin in turmeric, or the capsaicin in chilis.[19,20] Some herbs and spices, including paprika, rosemary, ginger, and turmeric, protect against DNA breaks and reduce inflammatory biomarkers.[21] Cumin, cinnamon, and clove have been studied for their antioxidant properties.[22] Some of the common Mediterranean spices, like rosemary and oregano, have been shown to be anti-inflammatory, antihyperlipidemic, antihypertensive, and antidiabetic.[23,24]

Some dried spices, like coriander seed, cumin seed, and fennel seed, may benefit from toasting for a few seconds in a dry skillet, while others, like cumin seed, curry leaves, dried red chilies, and mustard seed, may need to be tempered in hot oil for less than a minute to wake them up. Adding spice to food can make your dishes sing and allow you to decrease the amount of salt you may otherwise add to a dish.

Here are some common spice profiles:

Italian: basil, marjoram, oregano, rosemary, sage, thyme

Moroccan: cumin, cardamom, coriander, fenugreek, mint, saffron, ginger, vanilla

Turkish/Greek: mint, sumac, oregano, fennel, citrus, anise, cinnamon, dill, fenugreek, garlic, parsley, sesame, za'atar, Aleppo pepper

Indian: garlic, ginger, coriander, turmeric, asafedita, cinnamon, fenugreek, cardamom, mustard, clove, curry leaf, allspice, cumin

Mexican: cilantro, chili, cumin, coriander, garlic

Thai: basil, galangal, lemongrass, cilantro, coriander, ginger, lemongrass,

Japanese: garlic, ginger, sesame, scallion

Chinese: star anise, fennel, cinnamon, cloves, pepper, chili

Culinary Tip

Sometimes, we'll mix our own spices for a rub, but other times, we may use a premade spice rub on vegetables or fish before roasting or grilling. We'll put a rub designated for chicken on cauliflower and carrots, or a vegetable rub on a white fish. Feel free to mix and match and ignore what it was originally marketed for. Just be sure to read the label for any hidden sugars!

Pistachio Chia Pudding (V, VG, DF, GF)

Prep time: 10 minutes
Chill time: 2+ hours
Total time: 2 hours, 10 minutes

Yield: *4 servings*

3 tablespoons chia seeds
¾ cup plant-based milk
¾ teaspoon vanilla extract
½ cup pomegranate seeds
   (from 1 medium fruit)
1 tablespoon pistachios,
   chopped

Chia pudding makes a great breakfast or snack any time of day. In this easy recipe, you are getting seeds, nuts, and fruit. Pomegranates not only look extravagant, but their taste and texture will intrigue your taste buds. We store the pudding in small jars and bring it to work for an afternoon snack. If pomegranate is not in season, use blueberries or another fruit for extra antioxidants. Additional flavor options include lemon, ginger, cacao, or orange zest.

1. In a small bowl or mason jar, combine chia seeds, milk, and vanilla extract.
2. Cover and refrigerate for 2 hours or overnight.
3. Stir, then layer the mixture in a glass with pomegranate seeds just before serving.
4. Top with pistachios.

Olivia's Story

At twenty-seven years old and recently married, Olivia was already thinking about trying to conceive but was worried because, with the stress from her work at a high-tech company, she had started skipping every other cycle. She'd also put on ten pounds in the last four months even though she was eating well.

A month after her wedding, she decided to go to a fertility clinic for an evaluation. Her friends said she was nuts for going to a fertility clinic when she was so young and hadn't been trying to conceive for very long. They thought of a fertility clinic as a place to go only when you needed IVF, after many years of struggle. Olivia ignored them. She wanted to take charge and reverse the trends she had been seeing. Her history and blood tests supported a diagnosis of PCOS. Her doctor encouraged lifestyle changes and offered medications to help with ovulation. She wanted to try a natural approach first.

She quit her high-stress job because she felt that it was hurting her health, and she began consulting work instead. The flexible schedule gave her more time to shop and cook and attend regular exercise classes. With her diet, she started off doing what she read online, following a low-carb diet and counting calories. She quickly lost six pounds and felt great, but then she hit a plateau. Calorie counting wasn't working anymore.

After about six months, Olivia entered our Food for Fertility class, where she learned how to eat for fertility instead of weight loss. She learned that she did not need to be afraid of whole grains or fruits and began adding these food groups back into her diet.

She lost another five pounds during the class after she stopped counting calories and started eating more carbohydrates.

Whereas before, Olivia said she and her husband might eat a handful of vegetables, now they cooked twice as much. Instead of one bag of brussels sprouts, she would cook two. They made sure that half of the volume of food on their plates was vegetables. She always made sure to include some leafy greens and different varieties of nuts, and they would have a piece of fruit after dinner for something sweet.

She said she had more energy, her skin cleared up, and she was sleeping better. "I felt so much better," Olivia recalled. "I just thought I was a lethargic person, but I felt like a different human!" Her cycles began to change, becoming more regular. Instead of every other month, they shortened to every thirty-five days.

Three months later, her husband James said that Olivia looked a little different and wanted her to take a pregnancy test. She was hesitant because she didn't want to ruin her day with another negative test, but she agreed to take it. Two lines showed up right away. She was in shock; all of her hard work had paid off. She went on to have a healthy baby and conceived naturally two more times by sticking with her healthy habits!

Takeaways

1. Omega-3 fatty acids are nutritional superstars. There are three omega-3s: DHA, EPA, and ALA. They increase fertility by providing antioxidants, reducing inflammation, and improving metabolic health. They are also key supporters of brain health and neurological health.

2. Omega-6 fatty acids can be inflammatory and cause health problems in high quantities.

3. Vegetable oil used for restaurant foods, fast foods, processed foods, and fried foods contains a very high percentage of inflammatory omega-6 fatty acids.

4. Animal-based saturated fats from red meat, processed meats, and cheese can increase the risk of metabolic disease, dementia, and cancer and have a negative impact on fertility.

5. All nuts and seeds have multiple minerals, vitamins, fiber, and healthy fats.

6. Selenium, which is good for sperm and eggs, is highly concentrated in Brazil nuts.

7. Spices add flavor and antioxidants to your cooking.

Sample SMART Goals

1. When using oils for cooking at home, choose oils with a higher percentage of omega-3s, like olive oil or avocado oil. Cold-pressed oils are favored for their higher levels of micronutrients.
2. Aim to increase MUFA and PUFA intake from fatty fish and plants like avocados, olives, nuts, and seeds, and limit saturated fat from animal sources such as processed meat, red meat, and cheese.
3. Limit eating out to one to two times per week to reduce exposure to omega-6 fatty acids and saturated fats.
4. Limit fried foods and snack foods to reduce exposure to inflammatory omega-6 fatty acids.
5. Snack on a handful (about one ounce) of nuts or seeds daily.
6. Experiment with spices in your cooking.

Chapter 10

Food First, Supplements Second

Test Your Knowledge

Taking enough supplements can make up for an unhealthy diet. True/False
*Healthy sperm will improve fertility.** True/False

You've shifted your diet toward more plants, and you're now eating better to support your fertility. Congratulations! Not only is plant-forward eating good for fertility and your future pregnancy, but it will lower your risk of many diseases that strike people in their middle years such as diabetes, hypertension, heart disease, and certain cancers. Following a plant-forward diet can also reduce the severity of infections like COVID-19 and reduce the risk of developing autoimmune diseases and dementia. People who cook at home typically use higher quality ingredients, save money, and

---

* False. There is no one supplement that can provide you with every micronutrient your body needs to sustain itself. A prenatal supplement can support your fertility and prepare you for pregnancy, but a healthy diet is also necessary to meet your needs.

** True. Males are half of the equation for conception. Sperm from healthy men are higher quality. Luckily, men continue to create new sperm throughout their lives, so changes in lifestyle today can help over the upcoming months.

show less weight gain and diabetes over time.[1] Another benefit to consuming more plants is sustainability. By eating lower on the food chain, you are reducing deforestation and carbon emissions. This benefits everyone on our planet.

You are now familiar with all the components of the Food-First Fertility Plan: vegetables, fruits, beans, lentils, soy, whole grains, fish, and healthy fats. As you incorporate more fertility-promoting foods, you will reduce insulin resistance and inflammation, getting more energy in return. Shifting to incorporate more plants is a habit you can build up over time. Making food taste delicious is why we focus on the culinary aspect. You can also follow your adventurous spirit and adapt traditional family recipes to include more nutritious ingredients.

We've recommended you aim for eight servings of fruits and veggies per day, which means including them at most meals and snacks. Decide what vegetables you want to start with, then build your meal from there. Plants are also the root of the diet, literally, when it comes to protein. Legumes, including beans and lentils, are the protein backbone of a plant-forward diet and should be eaten most days to support your gut microbiome and reproductive health. Tofu, tempeh, and edamame from soybeans are good protein-packed, fertility-enhancing additions. From the animal category, fatty fish, pasture-raised eggs, and whole-fat yogurt round out the best fertility-promoting protein choices every week. For intake of other animal proteins, choose small portions of high-quality, grass-fed or pasture-raised animals for the most nutrient density. Include whole grains most days. Limit processed grains, ultra-processed foods, excess sugar, and artificial sweeteners. Pick your staples and enjoy them faithfully.

Vitamins and Supplements

Now, what about vitamins and supplements? It would be nice if we could get everything we need nutritionally from a pill, but unfortunately, this is not the case. We want you to first think about foods as wonderful delivery sources for most of the micro and macronutrients you'll need. Supplements come second.

Vitamins and supplements may be trying to treat deficiencies in your diet, but if there is a food source of a micronutrient, it will always be better than a pill. Take, for instance, vitamin C. Many people know that vitamin C is an antioxidant and helps the immune system. So, the idea that taking vitamin C could help prevent the common cold makes sense. You want to have a strong immune system, right? But many larger studies have now disproven this theory.[2] At best, vitamin C may shorten the symptoms from a cold by a few hours. There is no benefit to supplementing vitamin C for immunity, yet many people continue to use it anyway. Eating an orange or some slices of a red pepper would be a much better choice if you're looking to support your immune system with vitamin C.

Also keep in mind that vitamins and supplements work all over the body and rarely have isolated functions, so although you may see a benefit in one area of the body from increasing your intake of a vitamin or other supplement, too much may cause a problem in another. It would be nearly impossible to get too much of an individual micronutrient from carrots, cabbage, or raspberries, but you can get too much from a vitamin or supplement. Therefore, we recommend using vitamins and supplements with caution, and typically with a very specific purpose—such as during preconception and pregnancy. These are times when vitamins may prevent certain complications, like reducing the risk of neural tube defects (NTDs) in the fetus or helping to support fetal growth and development. In this chapter, we will delve into the research and discuss how you can complement your diet with a few vitamins and supplements, knowing that the data to support their use may be suboptimal.[3]

The data we have on vitamins and supplements is limited compared to the rigor of traditional pharmaceutical studies. When we look at human studies of vitamins and supplements, most of the studies have very small participant numbers. Although a positive benefit may be noted among a smaller group, the effect may be diminished in the larger population. And as some studies have shown, there could be downstream harmful effects that initially go unrecognized. Vitamins, supplements, and some hormones such as dehydroepiandrosterone (DHEA) and melatonin are not regulated by the FDA like prescription pharmaceuticals, which means there is less quality control. One way to ensure you are purchasing the highest-quality vitamins is to look for a third-party quality assurance label, especially for some of the more specialized supplements. Some companies pay a third party such as NSF, USP, or CL to inspect and test products for purity and content, and then place the third-party stamp on their label. This is the best way to ensure that you are getting the unadulterated vitamin or supplement you think you are getting, as well as the dosage listed on the label.

Next, we'll go over the main vitamins and supplements for everyone to consider, and then discuss some recommendations for special groups.

Vitamins and Supplements

	Recommended or Optional?	What does it do?
Folic acid	Recommended	Reduces risk of neural tube defects in fetus
Prenatal vitamin (PNV)	Recommended	Provides folic acid, iodine, vitamin B12, iron
Vitamin D	Recommended for those with deficiency	Works as a steroid hormone, supports ovulation, helps bone remodeling, reduces risk of some pregnancy complications
Antioxidants	Optional	May improve pregnancy rates
CoQ10	Optional	Supports mitochondrial energy production
Vitamin B12	Recommended for those who are plant-based	Supports DNA production, cell metabolism, nerve function, red blood cell formation

	Recommended or Optional?	What does it do?
Iron	Recommended for those who have a deficiency or are plant-based	Supports red blood cell production
Zinc	Recommended for those who are plant-based	Supports cell division, cell growth, immune system
Choline	Recommended for women who don't eat eggs or meat	Reduces risk of neural tube defects and aids in fetal brain development
DHA	Recommended for those who don't eat fish	Supports brain and neurological health
Inositol	Optional for those with PCOS	Improves insulin sensitivity, may help ovulation

Folic Acid

As you may recall, folic acid is the synthetic form of folate, a B vitamin important for cell growth. Women planning pregnancy should start taking 400 micrograms (mcg) of folic acid daily at least three months prior to pregnancy and during the first three months of pregnancy to reduce the risk of neural tube defects (NTD). Research has shown that a higher dose of folic acid, between 800 and 1,000 mcg, may have the added benefit of possibly reducing miscarriages.[4] Women at higher risk of neural tube defects should take 4 milligrams (4,000 mcg) of folic acid per day for three months prior to pregnancy and until the twelfth week of pregnancy. This includes women who have had a prior pregnancy with NTD, those at risk for NTD, and those with diabetes or malabsorption disorders, and those on certain anti-seizure medications.[5,6,7] Women with commonly occurring methylenetet-rahydrofolate reductase (MTHFR) gene mutations should take regular or higher folic acid supplementation—they do not need to take methylated form of folic acid.[8]

Prenatal Vitamins

In the United States, women who are trying to conceive are advised to take a prenatal vitamin (PNV), which includes the commonly recommended dose of folic acid. Keep in mind, some PNVs give you everything in one pill. Others divide up the dosage, so you have to take multiple pills throughout the day. Personally, we recommend the PNV that you only take once a day. This is easier and usually less expensive.

Not all PNVs are created equal. Prenatal gummies, among other types, may be missing key vitamins or minerals, such as iron. Only about half of manufactured PNVs contain enough iodine, which is important to support thyroid function, so be sure to read the label.[9] Vitamin B12 supports DNA production, and levels of B12 frequently run low for those eating mainly plants. Because iron is needed to build red blood cells, you don't want to start pregnancy with iron deficiency or anemia. Vitamin D deficiency is common, and many people need more than 400 IU daily. We recommend your preconception PNV contains these minimum amounts:

Folic acid	800 mcg
Vitamin B12	2.4 mcg
Vitamin D	400 IU
Iodine	150 mg
Iron	18 mcg
DHA	300 mg

The EARTH pro-fertility study showed that women who took higher doses of folic acid (>800 mcg/day), vitamin B12 (>15.8 mcg/day), and vitamin D3 (>843 IU/day) had higher pregnancy rates than those taking standard levels found in a PNV.[10] But many PNVs do not contain these higher amounts; you may choose to take separate supplements in addition to your regular PNV.

Vitamin D

We've mentioned vitamin D and the ways it can support health and fertility (see the Nutritional Spotlight on page 106). Having enough vitamin D may improve fertility and IVF outcomes,[11,12] and inadequate vitamin D levels have been associated with miscarriage.[13] The Cochrane Database of Systematic Reviews, the leading database for systematic reviews in health care, found that Vitamin D supplementation during pregnancy was also shown to reduce the risk of pre-eclampsia and gestational diabetes.[14]

Some people have low vitamin D levels year-round, while others become deficient in the winter months. We recommend getting your level checked at your doctor's office and supplementing if it is deficient. Aim for levels above 30 nanograms per milliliter (ng/mL) while trying to conceive and during pregnancy.

Antioxidants

Although antioxidants from foods are proven to be beneficial for fertility, most antioxidant supplements are of limited value. There are several antioxidants—N-acetylcysteine, melatonin, L-arginine, myo-inositol, carnitine, selenium, vitamin E, vitamin B complex, vitamin C, vitamin D plus calcium, and omega-3-polyunsaturated fatty acids—that have been examined in studies to see if they improve fertility. The Cochrane Database of Systematic Reviews looked at the effect of these antioxidants on male and female subfertility and found that most of the studies on this topic are too small and haven't had enough participants to tell if there is a benefit. More studies are needed on antioxidant supplements before they can be widely recommended.[15,16]

Coenzyme Q10

Coenzyme Q10 (CoQ10) is a naturally occurring antioxidant that has been studied more than others. It works with adenosine triphosphate (ATP) in the mitochondria to help with energy production and cell division. CoQ10 is present at higher levels in our bodies during youth and early adulthood, and then starts to naturally decline.

In the aging oocyte, oxidative stress and mitochondrial dysfunction can lead to higher rates of aneuploid (unbalanced chromosomes) embryos. Supplementation with CoQ10 has been proposed for women in their mid-thirties and older to reduce DNA damage and restore mitochondrial function associated with aging oocytes.[17]

Studies in older mice showed that CoQ10 supplementation for twelve to sixteen weeks made their eggs behave like they were from younger mice.[18] Unfortunately, the equivalent duration in humans would be about ten years of exposure! A recent small meta-analysis on CoQ10 supplementation combined five studies to look at the supplement's impact on IVF outcomes and again, the data wasn't totally supportive. Although CoQ10 supplementation may help reduce oxidative stress and mitochondrial dysfunction, so far it hasn't shown an increase in live birth outcomes.[19,20] Still, many women trying to conceive choose to supplement with CoQ10 due to the potential benefits. For men, CoQ10 has been shown to increase the three main sperm parameters—count, motility, and morphology—when taking CoQ10 supplementation for six months or longer.[21,22]

Vitamins and Supplements for Special Groups

A couple of groups may benefit from some additional vitamins and supplements in addition to a PNV. This includes individuals who are almost exclusively eating plants and women with PCOS.

Plant-Centric Eaters

Of course, we advocate for everyone to eat a plant-forward, whole-food diet to support fertility. However, if you are exclusively plant-based, that is, you don't incorporate eggs, fish, or small portions of meat into your diet, then you may be at risk for micronutrient deficiencies, most commonly vitamin B12, iron, zinc, choline, and omega-3s. Vitamin B12 is found mainly in animal foods, but it is also found naturally on some produce grown in the ground and in nutritional yeast. Because B vitamins are water soluble, your body cannot store them, so they need to be replenished frequently. Your body needs about 2.4 micrograms of vitamin B12 daily.

Iron is an essential mineral that is important in the production of red blood cells and prevention of anemia. It comes mainly from animal and plant sources such as organ meat, red meat, shellfish, spinach, legumes, and some seeds. Prenatal vitamins may contain adequate iron, but some women do not absorb iron well and may need additional supplementation. While trying to conceive, 18 milligrams of iron daily is recommended, with 27 milligrams per day recommended during pregnancy.

Zinc is important for cell division and growth. It is included in some PNV but not others. The naturally occurring sources of zinc include nuts, seeds, whole grains, legumes, seafood, and red meat. Those who are mainly plant-based may not get enough zinc from foods and may benefit from a PNV or supplement that includes 15 milligrams of zinc.

An essential nutrient, choline is important for egg development. Choline is produced in your body in small amounts and is also found in eggs, dairy, animal proteins, and cruciferous vegetables. Choline works together with folic acid to prevent neural tube defects and aids in fetal brain development. It also can help improve insulin resistance and fatty liver. Look for choline in your PNV and consider supplementing 350 milligrams of choline bitartrate daily if you have minimal amounts coming from animal foods.

Some PNVs include 300 milligrams of DHA, an omega-3 fatty acid that supports fetal brain and neurological development. If your PNV doesn't include DHA, and you don't eat fish, then plan to take around 300 milligrams per day of a DHA supplement. This may be sold as fish oil, krill oil, or algal oil.

Women with PCOS

PCOS is one of the most common causes of infertility because regular ovulation does not occur. Some women with PCOS may choose to take additional vitamins and supplements to support their health such as myoinositol, vitamin D, iron, and B12. Inositols are naturally occurring sugars that can help regulate cycles, improve egg quality and ovulation potential, and reduce insulin resistance, which may be particularly beneficial for women with PCOS.[23] Myoinositol, or a combination of myoinositol and D-chiro-inositol, may be taken to help reduce insulin resistance and improve ovulation in women with PCOS. Until more data is available, we recommend discontinuing inositol supplementation with pregnancy.

Many of the other vitamins we've discussed in this chapter as being beneficial for fertility are also helpful for women with PCOS. For women with PCOS, vitamin D supplementation may improve many metabolic parameters such as glucose levels, insulin sensitivity, triglycerides, and hormone levels.[24] Some women with PCOS may have iron deficiency and may benefit from supplementation.[25] CoQ10 has also been shown to decrease some inflammatory markers and improve glucose and lipid metabolism in some women with PCOS.[26] Finally, some women with PCOS may develop vitamin B12 deficiency if they take the prescription medication metformin. Metformin is prescribed to treat type 2 diabetes and help decrease insulin resistance, and it can decrease intestinal absorption of vitamin B12. If you take this medication, ask to have your B12 level checked.

———

In summary, we want you to get most of your micronutrients from food. Some vitamins and supplements may be good additions while trying to conceive, but others have limited data to support their use. It's worth mentioning here that Chinese herbs prescribed by Traditional Chinese Medicine physicians may also be used to treat infertility, but we have not mentioned any Chinese herbs or other herbs here because they are beyond our scope of expertise.

Be sure to discuss any medications, vitamins, supplements, herbs, and over-the-counter hormones with your health care provider. Fertility physicians will want to know what you are taking and may recommend you discontinue some of these prior to an IVF cycle and during pregnancy. Prenatal vitamins may be safely continued throughout fertility treatments and during pregnancy.

Jessica's Story

Jessica had tried to conceive naturally for four years. Her cycles were very regular, but she had not had a single positive pregnancy test. She decided to see a fertility physician at age thirty-three. All of her testing came back normal, other than a mild male factor. She and her partner tried two intrauterine inseminations, but these were unsuccessful.

Looking for that magic bullet that could help, she requested a referral for acupuncture and nutrition counseling, and these became her support pillars. She wound up in our Food for Fertility class and found it to be a valuable experience. "I knew that my diet wasn't the best and I wanted to get ideas, be inspired, and learn how to cook healthier food," Jessica said. "I had a skill gap—I didn't know how to make healthy food taste good. I had negative associations with food and health.

"Learning how food helps fertility was very useful. I preferred to focus on food before supplements, although I took the ones I needed," she added. Jessica took the class twice, to reinforce her skills and habits. "The first time I took the class I was being more consistent, but I started to slip. I wanted to come back to build skills at a deeper level. I wanted the positive habits to become automatic," she recalled.

"One of the things I found that really helps is meal planning and prepping," Jessica continued. "It sets the tone for the week. If I have a plan, I'm less likely to call Uber Eats. I learned how to use beans to make food more filling. I'll add them to Mexican dishes or have them as a side instead of rice. We like pinto beans, but also cannellini beans and black beans. We make pintos from scratch—the others we buy in cans. We eat them weekly. We have a few meals we really like: the white bean chili chicken, and salad with black beans, cilantro, and cumin-rubbed chicken on the side."

After so many years of struggle, Jessica ultimately conceived. "What I learned during fertility treatments was so helpful. I added vegetables to smoothies. I had no diabetes and managed my hypertension during pregnancy. For sure, the class taught me good habits with vegetables—learning how to add them to soups and other dishes. Some of my favorites were brussels sprouts and roasted vegetables. One of my goals is always to have one fruit and vegetable at each meal. That helps keep me on track. It is so simple but helps!"

Jessica gained confidence over time with her cooking skills and comfort around food. "I had to let go of dieting and restriction," she told us. She also embraced techniques to reduce her stress and practices positive self-care now with affirmations and mindfulness. "I found mindful eating helped me be more aware of what I was eating, and not overeat. These were the things that held it together for me." Her habits seem to have stuck!

Takeaways

1. Almost all your nutrients can come from food. Make eating more plant-based foods easy by having fresh produce available and keeping a well-stocked pantry.
2. For women trying to conceive, prenatal vitamins and folic acid are recommended at least three months prior to pregnancy and during pregnancy. Some supplements, however, should be discontinued while trying to conceive and with pregnancy.
3. Those eating a mainly plant-based diet should consider supplementing iron, choline, vitamin B12, and DHA.
4. Women with PCOS may benefit from extra vitamin D and insulin sensitizers such as inositol.

Sample SMART Goals

1. Review the label of your PNV and other supplements to confirm they contain what you need.
2. Think about whether you may be low in certain micronutrients like vitamin D, vitamin B12, choline, iron, and DHA/EPA— consider asking for a blood test from your doctor to confirm adequate levels of vitamin D, vitamin B12, and ferritin. Supplement if levels of a given nutrient are low, or if you do not take in enough through food sources.
3. Look to purchase higher-quality supplements that have been third-party certified.

Chapter 11

The Fertility Boosters

Move More, Stress Less, and Sleep Well

n this chapter, we're going to discuss a few lifestyle activities that can work to boost your fertility. They include physical activity, stress reduction, and restorative sleep. If you establish some good habits that work for you, you'll improve your metabolism, decrease inflammation, improve hormonal balance, reduce anxiety and depressive symptoms, and shorten your time to pregnancy.

Move More

Test Your Knowledge
Strength training will just bulk me up.* True/False
Cardio exercise must be at least an hour to improve my health.** True/False

---

* False. Benefits of weight training include increased strength, increased energy, improved mood, reduced stress, reduced risk of injury, and management of chronic health issues like diabetes.

** False. There are so many benefits for cardio workouts! The CDC recommends at least 150 minutes of moderate-intensity physical activity weekly, 75 minutes vigorous activity each week, or some combination. It is fine to break up cardio into 10-minute intervals.

Our bodies are meant to move. Because physical activity has so many health benefits, it should really be part of everyone's daily routine. Moving enhances positive emotions and causes immediate enjoyment. Neuroscience tells us that exercise activates neurotransmitters like endorphins, dopamine, serotonin, and endocannabinoids. These neurotransmitters tell us when something is pleasurable and, in turn, deliver motivation and make us feel more hopeful. Exercise can help a person deal with stress and sensitizes the brain to experiences involving pleasure and joy. It enhances the robustness of our reward system, the system that motivates you to expect good things to happen. Certainly, you need hope and a robust reward system when you are trying to conceive.

In addition to lifting our mood, physical activity improves our metabolism. It decreases insulin resistance, stabilizes weight, and reduces the risk of developing type 2 diabetes. And exercising doesn't have to mean going to the gym to sweat for an hour. Activity can be light, moderate, or intense. It can be as short as a ten-minute walk after a meal, or as long as a multi-hour hike. And finally, some types of aerobic exercise, at moderate or high intensity, can provide an even more intense feeling of bliss known as the runner's high for some people. The good news is that this feeling can occur with multiple types of exercise, so substitute your favorite activity here!

Advantages to Exercise

Improved fertility (see next section!)

Improved mood

More positive emotions

Increased social connectedness

Improved mental clarity and focus

Improved memory and learning

Improved insulin sensitivity

Reduced stress

Weight stabilization

Reduced risk of type 2 diabetes and dementia

Improved longevity

Exercise and Fertility

Physical activity can also boost your fertility, but it's a bit of a Goldilocks scenario. You don't want to do so much exercise that you shut down your hormones that control reproduction, but you also don't want to do so little that you slow down your metabolism. For most people, that translates to about thirty to sixty minutes of moderate activity daily. We recommend individualizing it based on your daily routine. If you are someone on your feet running around all day, you may already be meeting your activity goals. But if you have a sedentary job and are working at a computer for eight hours a day, then sixty minutes of some physical activity (it's okay to break it up into two or three smaller sessions) is recommended. For many women with PCOS who have insulin resistance, more time spent being physically active can help ovulation to occur more often, and pregnancy to occur naturally. Research shows that staying active improves fertility for most women and shortens time to pregnancy, so you want to make sure you have some good physical activity built into your daily routine.[1,2]

Exercise and the Menstrual Cycle

While most women have no change in ovulation or their menstrual pattern with regular daily exercise, some women with irregular cycles (particularly those with PCOS) can benefit from more exercise to initiate ovulation, while some women with absent menstrual cycles—particularly those with relative energy deficiency in sport (RED-S), or hypothalamic amenorrhea—can benefit from reducing exercise to restore ovulation. We advise anyone with irregular or absent cycles to speak with a dietitian or nutritionist and a reproductive endocrinologist for further testing and treatment.

Exercise and PCOS

We've mentioned PCOS (polycystic ovary syndrome) previously. It is one of the most common causes of infertility, as women with PCOS do not release an egg every month. They also have higher insulin resistance. By reducing insulin resistance with moderate-intensity exercise for around sixty minutes daily or high-intensity exercise for thirty minutes daily, natural ovulation may resume and conception is more likely to follow.[3] High-intensity interval training (HIIT) has also been shown to improve insulin resistance and restore ovulation in women with PCOS.[4] Resistance training or strength training also improves insulin sensitivity and ovulation.[5] The exact mechanism for how insulin resistance contributes to anovulation is not well understood, but it is great news that both aerobic and resistance training can increase ovulation and natural conception for women with PCOS.

Exercise and RED-S

For some women, too much exercise, in either intensity or duration, can exert a negative effect on reproductive hormones if they are not nourishing their bodies appropriately. Women participating in moderate to intense exercise for too many hours per week without adequate energy intake can develop infertility by interrupting the hypothalamic pituitary ovary axis and disrupting ovulation.[6] This can lead to hypothalamic amenorrhea, or absent menses from a lack of hormonal signaling coming from the hypothalamus.

Any woman exercising for many hours and not meeting energy needs through nutrition may experience disruption in her menstrual cycles, regardless of her size. This condition is called relative energy deficiency in sport (RED-S). For women who enjoy frequent, intense exercise, if menstrual cycles are regular, there is likely nothing to worry about. However, for strenuous exercisers, if cycles are irregular or absent, it is possible that more energy intake is needed to meet the demands of exercise. The book *No Period, Now What?* by Nicola Rinaldi, PhD,[7] is a good resource to learn more about hypothalamic amenorrhea for runners and athletes.

Exercise Zones

Exercise can be categorized into one of five different levels (or zones) based on your level of exertion or, more precisely, the percentage of your age-based maximum heart rate:

- Zone 1 is very light intensity, at 50 to 60 percent of your max heart rate.
- Zone 2 is light intensity, at 60 to 70 percent of your max heart rate.
- Zone 3 is moderate intensity, at 70 to 80 percent of your max heart rate.
- Zone 4 is hard intensity, at 80 to 90 percent of your max heart rate.
- Zone 5 is maximum activity, at 90 to 100 percent of your max heart rate.

One way to estimate your target heart rate in different zones is to calculate your age-based maximum heart rate. Subtract your age from 220. For instance, at age thirty, you would calculate your maximum heart rate (max HR) to be 190 (220–30). Then multiply by the percentages for a given range. So, for zone 2, your heart rate would be in the range of 114 to 133 beats per minute.

Light-intensity exercise, or zone 2, is rated at about a 3 to 4 out of 10 on the effort scale and takes advantage of a slower pace for longer duration. It is frequently considered the level for endurance exercise. You would not sound out of breath if you were carrying on a conversation at this level and you're unlikely to break a sweat. You can get enough oxygen by breathing through your nose. It can include activities like brisk walking, biking, or swimming. Moderate intensity, or zone 3 exercise, means you're putting out an effort of about 5 to 6 out of 10 and will likely break a sweat after about ten minutes. It's the pace of a walk up a hill or a jog. You can carry on a conversation with someone walking next to you, but you don't have enough energy to belt out a song as you could if you were standing still. Vigorous or hard exercise, or zone 4, has you working at a level of around 7 or 8 out of 10, where you are feeling out of breath and could not carry on a conversation. For vigorous exercise, less time is needed for the same aerobic benefit. Fifteen minutes a day, or seventy-five minutes a week, gives you the same benefit as thirty minutes of moderate exercise per day.

That being said, it's a good idea to emphasize movement in zone 2. An advantage is that zone 2 exercise conditions your mitochondria,[8] the organelles in your cell that provide energy for cell division. We know how important mitochondria are for reproduction and embryo development! This is why an hour in zone 2 every day may be a good idea for reproduction and long-term metabolic health.

For additional cardiovascular conditioning, thirty to sixty minutes in zone 3 or up to twenty minutes in zone 4 may be okay while trying to conceive naturally. Avoid spending time at the highest level (zone 5) unless you are well conditioned.

If you are participating or preparing for an active IVF cycle, the recommendation may be to reduce your exercise intensity and stick to zone 2. If you have any questions about how much exercise you should do, or if you have any pre-existing medical conditions, discuss it with your health care provider before starting.

Exercise outdoors (green exercise) provides even more of a mood boost than exercise indoors. Breathing fresh air, getting sunlight, and enjoying nature, even in a city park, can decrease depressive symptoms.[9,10] Forest bathing, or shinrin-yoku, which is taking in the outdoor green space using all our senses, confers even more benefits, temporarily reducing cortisol levels, heart rate, and blood pressure.[11,12] How much time in nature do you need to get the benefits? Well, a group of investigators looked at that question and found that at least 120 minutes a week outdoors is associated with positive benefits. This could be a twenty-minute walk every day in a city park, or a two-hour hike on the weekend.[13]

Walking is one of the easiest forms of exercise, and integrated technology has made counting steps a simple way to measure your activity. If you would like a target, we recommend aiming for about 6,000 steps per day for a mood lift, or greater than 7,000 for overall health and longevity. The 10,000-steps target was coined in 1965 as a marketing tool—you don't actually have to hit 10,000 steps as most health benefits have been observed at lower step counts. Of course, if you prefer to pursue other forms of activity like yoga, gardening, spin class, or golfing, we think that's great, too! Whatever gets you moving is a good thing.

Resistance Training

Adding two or three sessions a week of ten-minute resistance training in addition to aerobic activity can improve insulin resistance and may help your fertility even further. Resistance or strength training uses your body weight, exercise bands, free weights, or weight machines to strengthen different muscle groups. Examples include squats, lunges, push-ups, and core-strengthening exercises. Functional movements like lifting and gentle twisting, balancing, and stretching also benefit our bodies and become increasingly important as we age.

Make Movement a Habit

Some people think that if they can't make it to the gym for an hour, why bother? Well, bother you should! For someone who doesn't exercise regularly, a short walk can spark your motivation. Start by committing to something simple like a walk around the block. One block can stretch to two, then three, and soon, you're walking a mile. Once you start moving, the positive mood boost you'll experience will increase your motivation and make you more likely to continue. It doesn't take much time to get a benefit. Just fifteen minutes of walking after meals has been shown to improve insulin resistance and reduce the risk of diabetes.[14]

Put It on Your Calendar!

Distractions are a part of life, so set your intention for exercise like you would any other important task. Write an exercise prescription for yourself and include the type of exercise, the duration, location, and intensity. For instance, schedule a brisk walk outside for ten minutes in the morning, ten minutes after lunch, and twenty minutes after dinner. From a behavioral standpoint, you can tie the activity to a reward like listening to music or a podcast, or catching up with a friend. Behaviorist Katy Milkman has called this "temptation bundling," where you tie something a little more difficult to something highly rewarding.[15] Once you develop a habit, you may be surprised with how good you start to feel.

Intuitive Movement

Taking an intuitive approach to your habits doesn't just apply to eating; you can apply the same principles to physical activity. How does your body enjoy moving? Walking outside and breathing fresh air? Yoga? Dancing in the kitchen? Does riding a bike make you feel like a kid again? Take advantage of the activities that bring you the most joy. Ten to fifteen minutes of moving can make you feel good, improve insulin sensitivity, and reduce inflammation, thus boosting fertility. Embrace moving your body in a pleasurable way every day. You won't believe how quickly a thirty-minute walk goes by when you're catching up with a good friend. It's about learning to incorporate health-promoting behaviors to enhance your preconception time and future pregnancy.

Stress Less

Test Your Knowledge
Breathing exercises can help reduce my stress. True/False
*Stress can trigger binge eating.** True/False

Does stress cause infertility or does infertility cause stress?[16] This is a tough one to pin down. We don't think anyone would argue with the fact that dealing

---

* True. Changing how we breathe can change how we feel. Many methods are easy to learn and incredibly helpful.

** True. Your body produces cortisol when you are stressed, which in turn can increase hunger. When this happens, we are especially susceptible to sweets—sugar intake can lead to a release of the neuro hormones serotonin and dopamine, which can temporarily give us a mood boost but isn't a great long-term coping strategy.

with infertility causes stress, but some studies have shown that stress may increase infertility,[17] and experiencing stressful life events may contribute to lower success with fertility treatments.[18,19,20] The exact effect of stress on the reproductive system can be hard to assess because nothing occurs in isolation, but we know that stress can cause physical and emotional changes. Stress can cause activation of the sympathetic nervous system, the "fight or flight" pathway that can affect a person's health in negative ways. The sympathetic system causes heart rate and blood pressure to elevate, glucose to rise in the bloodstream, and the immune system to be activated. This response is important for the body if you are escaping from a predator, but bad for the body if chronically turned on. Clinical studies have shown how the relaxation response can improve medical conditions that are worsened by stress such as hypertension, pain, and infertility.

Psychological stress is increased in situations where you don't have control. This lack of control is one of the main stressors that comes from dealing with infertility. Struggling to conceive can put a strain on sexuality and intimacy, as timed intercourse becomes a prescribed duty every month.[21] And chronic stress can lead to erectile dysfunction or missed ovulation, further complicating fertility attempts.

If you are feeling more anxiety or depressive symptoms, realize this is common and strongly consider seeing a therapist or sharing your feelings with a close friend or family member. Try not to let these feelings stop you from moving forward.

We encourage you to have tools available to reduce your stress as you are trying to conceive or deal with any difficulties. Several of these techniques have been shown to lower stress for those facing difficult life situations, some specifically in the setting of infertility. Reducing stress prior to fertility treatments may reduce the number of treatments that are needed, or it may improve resiliency if treatments fail.[22] Some of these long-term interventions have been shown to increase pregnancy rates by about 20 percent for those undergoing assisted reproductive technologies like IVF.[23] Participation in mind-body programs that combine some of these tools and are led by trained mental health professionals across the country have resulted in lower rates of anxiety and depression, and possibly higher pregnancy rates.[24,25]

A few of these stress-reduction tools have been specifically studied for infertility patients. Expressive writing as a stress reduction tool has been looked at as a tool for couples with infertility. In one small study, emotional disclosure writing about fertility was found to decrease depressive symptoms.[26] In another small study out of China, practicing mindfulness was shown to be helpful for women going through their first IVF cycle.[27]

Tools to Reduce Stress

Cognitive behavioral therapy	Prayer
Mind-body programs	Exercise
Acupuncture	Deep breathing
Yoga	Time in nature
Expressive writing	Digital detox
Music therapy	Eating whole foods
Practicing gratitude	Positive self-talk
Meditation	Time with friends
Mindfulness	Laughing

The Importance of Resilience

Why is building resilience so important? Resilience is the ability to respond positively in the face of physical or psychological adversity. When you have practiced engaging in a positive, bounce-back mindset, you're better at adapting to life's challenges. It is another tool to help one adapt to acute or chronic stressors such as infertility.[28] Cultivating resilience will help you to endure the ups and downs of fertility treatments.

Breath Work and Mini Meditations

Mini meditations can also be helpful to manage stress, and you can do them throughout the day. If you don't have time for a twenty-minute meditation, take one minute to focus on your breathing. Breathing exercises can be deeply centering and relaxing.

Try box breathing as a first step. Close your eyes. Breathe to a slow count of four on your inhale, hold for four counts, exhale for four, wait for four, then repeat for five cycles. These mini meditations can engage the relaxation response, lower your heart rate and blood pressure, and allow you to focus more deeply at the task at hand. Give it a try!

Sleep Well

Test Your Knowledge

Chronic sleep deprivation can contribute to weight gain.* True/False
An afternoon coffee can disrupt your sleep.** True/False

Sleep plays a key role in our lives, allowing our bodies to recover from the day, consolidating memories, removing toxins, processing emotionally difficult events, and thinking up creative ideas. Many people do not realize how critically important sleep is for our day-to-day functioning and long-term health. Most adults need seven to nine hours of quality sleep to be fully recharged for

---

* True. When you're sleep deprived, you are more likely to feel tired and have low energy. In turn you may be reaching for quick energy like sodas or sweets and have less capacity to prepare meals.

** True. It's recommended to stop drinking caffeine at least ten hours before you plan to go to sleep. For most people, it's best to stop before noon.

the next day. Some individuals experience poor sleep due to obstructive sleep apnea or shift work. Others choose to restrict their sleep, believing it is not important, or use caffeine or alcohol, which can reduce sleep quality. Regardless of the reason, inadequate sleep can lead to a host of problems, including reduced fertility.

The metabolic downsides of sleep deprivation are numerous. It can lead to diabetes, hypertension, weight gain, and eventually heart disease.[29] Sleep deprivation can disturb the functioning of the gut microbiome and reduce the responsiveness of the immune system, making us more susceptible to infections.

Women with PCOS have higher rates of obstructive sleep apnea, which can add to poor sleep quality, interruption of hormone secretion, menstrual irregularity, anxiety, and depression.[30] Insulin resistance also increases the rates of sleep apnea in women with PCOS.[31,32] Not only is insulin resistance a risk factor for developing sleep apnea but sleep apnea can worsen insulin resistance and metabolic signals in women with PCOS.[33] According to the 2018 PCOS international guidelines, screening for obstructive sleep apnea is now recommended as part of routine care for women with PCOS.[34]

Poor sleep can also suppress estrogen and testosterone secretion, which can lower sex drive. Erectile dysfunction can worsen with poorer sleep. Men who sleep less than seven hours or more than eight hours per night appear to be at higher risk of infertility.[35] A similar observation was seen in women, where those sleeping more than nine hours or less than six hours showed lower pregnancy rates per cycle.[36] One bit of good news: having more sex, which many people do while trying to conceive, may help improve quality of sleep by increasing the hormone oxytocin during orgasm and decreasing cortisol levels.

Shorter sleep duration has been shown to have a negative effect on female fertility, male fertility, and IVF outcomes, so it is important that you strive for good sleep.[37] Changes in your hormones and stress can also disrupt sleep. In one survey, 35 percent of women experiencing infertility reported sleep disturbances.[38] Sleep quality negatively impacted outcomes as stress increased for women going through IVF treatment cycles.[39]

One study looked at sleep duration and quality for twenty-two women going through IVF cycles. It revealed that many had short sleep duration, higher daytime sleepiness, and poor sleep quality. There was a linear relationship between total sleep time and number of eggs retrieved. The average duration of sleep was 7.1 hours with a maximum sleep duration of 8.3 hours. Less than seven hours of sleep was noted in 45 to 70 percent of the women. More hours sleeping correlated with more eggs at egg retrieval.[40] How could this happen? Poor sleep duration, less than seven hours, could potentially lead to fewer eggs and lower egg quality by increasing activation of the sympathetic nervous system, neuroendocrine hormones, and cortisol.[41] In another survey of more than three thousand women, those who reported better sleep quality demonstrated a 12 percent higher live birth rate from IVF cycles.[42]

The effect of sleep disturbance on fertility is most dramatically illustrated for women who perform shift work. Working night shifts is known to disrupt sleep and predispose individuals to a wide range of disorders, including decreased fertility.[43] This can occur by altering female hormone secretion, increasing stress, and disrupting menstrual cycles.[44,45] In one observational study, female night shift workers younger than thirty-five years old were more likely to need fertility treatments and have menstrual irregularities or endometriosis than women who worked daytime hours.[46] Shift work has also been associated with increased rates of miscarriage and preterm birth, although the reasons are not well understood.[47,48,49] We recommend women who work the night shift seek fertility treatments earlier than they otherwise would due to the recognized disruption on reproduction.

Tips for Sleeping Well

You'll notice that the advice for good sleep overlaps quite a bit with the tools for stress reduction. If you feel well rested and do not experience excessive daytime sleepiness, you are likely getting enough sleep. It is common for individuals to have occasional windows of disrupted sleep, but if you snore loudly or have persistent daytime sleepiness, we recommend you see a sleep medicine specialist. Getting enough sleep is critical to your health and fertility.

Ideas to Establish a Relaxing Nighttime Routine

Read a book

Journal: write a gratitude exercise or "to do" list for the next day

Practice yoga or meditation

Take a warm shower or bath

Listen to music

Discontinue screen use one to two hours prior to bedtime

Keep the bedroom for sleep and sex only

Keep the bedroom cool and dark

Establish a Consistent Daytime Routine

Follow a consistent wake/sleep schedule

Walk for ten to twenty minutes outside once the sun is up to reset your circadian clock

Exercise daily for good sleep at night

Limit caffeine to one cup before 10 AM

Avoid alcohol

Finish dinner three hours prior to bedtime

April's Story

At age fifteen, April's menstrual cycles stopped. Over the next fifteen years, she met with more than twenty doctors and followed every suggestion her providers offered to try to get her period back. Meanwhile, she walked four miles a day, participated in an extensive yoga practice, and ate a restrictive, low-calorie diet. In her mind, this was practicing a healthful lifestyle.

Once she started trying to conceive, no one ever suggested she reduce her activity or eat more to improve her reproductive health. She was always very open with her health care providers about how active she was and what she ate. Yoga and walking are great, they told her. April's thyroid and hormone levels were measured, and she was told they were low. One provider suggested an avocado every day. She tried their suggestions. Still no period, no pregnancy.

Her lack of success restoring her period prompted April to take the next step on her journey to conceive. She and her husband scheduled an assessment with a fertility doctor. During the intake, nothing was ever mentioned about her diet or exercise, maybe because she was thin. She asked the doctor if food could help her get pregnant, and they suggested a Mediterranean diet. April was never told that she might need to eat more, and her nutrition intake was never evaluated. The topic of available energy for fertility was never discussed.

April's first intrauterine insemination (IUI) cycle was canceled because she stimulated too many eggs, which would have put her at risk for triplets or higher. She moved on to an IVF cycle, which did not produce any normal embryos. Frustrated, she tried a different doctor and clinic, read many fertility wellness books, and followed their guidelines of no sugar and other specific diet restrictions. She had another IUI cycle, and this time, she had no response to the medications. She tried a second IVF cycle, which resulted in one embryo that was too weak to test or transfer—another failed cycle.

April and her husband decided to give up on fertility treatments and choose adoption. They were thrilled to bring home a beautiful new daughter. But after she became a mom, April felt even more strongly about wanting to have a normal period. She met with her original reproductive medicine doctor with a request of focusing on just getting a cycle. "I don't have to get pregnant, but I want my period." She was referred to a sports medicine doctor who specialized in metabolism.

During her intake blood work, she was diagnosed with extreme anorexia. She was referred to local eating disorder centers for immediate treatment. She learned that she had obsessive compulsive disorder (OCD) and was a very restrictive eater. She was not providing herself with enough available energy for her reproductive hormones to work as designed. They were shut down!

She decided to put together her own treatment team and began working with Judy for medical nutrition therapy for her anorexia nervosa. April learned how to trust herself to eat enough and gained more weight than she had been comfortable with in the past. She backed off on her exercise regimen. She gained some weight and liked the energy she felt, though she struggled some to get used to her larger body. She loved all the food she could finally give herself permission to eat. Bagels became her favorite; before, she had always restricted eating carbohydrates. Within a few months she "felt a little crazy, like maybe my hormones were turning on?"

All the doctors she'd seen had told April she had poor egg quality. Although she hadn't gotten a period, she found out she was eight weeks pregnant! She had ovulated and conceived when the first egg was released. "Eating and nourishing my body had everything to do with getting pregnant." She walked and did gentle yoga, but nothing excessive.

She was in disbelief that no one had previously asked or talked about food or exercise on her fertility journey. "It's not medicine, and it doesn't need a prescription, but I needed to know how to nourish my body." April had a wonderful pregnancy without complications and, soon thereafter, brought her second daughter home. In the years that followed the birth of her daughter, she kept up the skills she had learned to meet her nutritional needs and began having normal periods. Two years later, she conceived her son without any assistance.

Takeaways

1. Exercise improves mood, insulin resistance, and fertility.
2. Stress can negatively impact mental and physical health. Managing stress is important to improve fertility.
3. Sleep is crucial for our health and well-being.
4. Not getting enough sleep can lead to hormonal dysregulation and health problems, including reduced fertility.

Sample SMART Goals

1. Aim for sixty minutes of light-intensity exercise most days.
2. Aim for a weekly dose of nature: twenty minutes daily, or two hours weekly.
3. Schedule ten minutes of active movement after meals.
4. Break up sitting for extended periods of time with standing, stretching, and short walks.
5. Add resistance or body-weight exercises two to three times per week.
6. Pick a mindfulness exercise to try out.
7. Try a mini meditation breathing exercise.
8. Connect with a friend once a week, ideally in person.
9. Ask yourself if you are getting enough sleep. Challenge yourself to go to bed thirty minutes to an hour earlier and see if you feel more rested in the morning.
10. Enjoy a morning walk outside once the sun is up to reset your master circadian clock.

Chapter 12

Fertility Disruptors

Part 1: Ingestible Substances

Test Your Knowledge

Processed foods are more convenient. * True/False

It's okay to drink alcohol until you have a positive pregnancy test. ** True/False

We have focused thus far on the foods, supplements, and boosters that you should include on your path to parenthood. Now let's spend some time discussing things that may be taking up space in your life that aren't doing you any good and could, in fact, be disrupting your fertility. These include excess sugar, artificial sweeteners, alcohol, tobacco, cannabis, and caffeine.

---

* False. Home meal preparation, batch cooking, and planning can provide you with meals and snacks that are just as easy.

** False. Alcohol can decrease your fertility prior to pregnancy and is best avoided.

Added Sugars and Artificial Sweeteners

Added sugars in foods can cause glucose spikes, insulin resistance, and chronic inflammation, all of which can impair fertility. Different forms of sugar are frequently added to processed and ultra-processed foods and beverages to increase palatability. For example, did you know that a tablespoon of ketchup, which you probably don't consider to be a sweet food, contains 4 grams of added sugar?

Sugars come in many different forms, and they can be hard to detect on a food label. Most people are familiar with high-fructose corn syrup, but you can look for anything that ends in -ose or fructose, glucose, or sucrose. If you're curious, search for "hidden sugars on food labels" online and you can see how many names there are. It's quite remarkable! Also, food labels tell you how much added sugar is in the product per serving size. Examining labels is a good way to start to get a sense of your added sugar intake.

Beverages are a common source of added sugars. A 20-ounce soft drink can contain a whopping 65 grams of sugar, typically in the form of corn syrup—way over the daily recommended amount of 25 grams. Coffee shops, espresso stands, and bubble tea establishments are particularly common sources of hidden sugars. A 16-ounce vanilla latte has about 34 grams of added sugar and a 20-ounce milk bubble tea may have up to 100 grams of sugar—more than what's in a slice of cake! The added calories from these sugar-sweetened beverages can contribute to undesired weight gain and chronic health problems like diabetes and tooth decay.[1]

Diet drinks and artificial sweeteners were supposed to be the answer to replace all the added sugar in our foods and beverages, touted as giving us all the sweetness without the negative effects. But the diet cola that so many people seem to be addicted to may cause health problems as well. Although most artificial sweeteners have fewer calories than sugar, studies are now showing that people who consume artificial sweeteners may actually gain weight over time, as well as having an increased risk of metabolic disease. Why could this happen? When the body doesn't get the calories it expects from the sweet stimulus, it may drive the individual to consume more calories from other foods throughout the day.

One of the first studies to recognize that people who drank artificially sweetened beverages gained weight was the San Antonio Heart study.[2] Over seven to eight years, those who drank more diet drinks had more weight gain over time compared to those who didn't consume diet drinks. It was only a pound or two, but it challenged the idea that artificially sweetened beverages would help with weight loss. Since then, other studies have shown similar trends. People consuming artificial sweeteners tend not to lose weight and may even gain weight over time.

Both sugar and artificial sweeteners can trigger a dopamine release in your brain, boosting your mood and making you crave more sweetness to get the dopamine rise again. One common artificial sweetener, Splenda, or sucralose, is 400 to 700 times sweeter than natural sugar, without any calories. This conditions human taste buds to want more and more sweetness, a cycle that is hard to break.[3] If that's not enough of a problem, aspartame has recently been called out by the World Health Organization (WHO) as possibly carcinogenic.[4]

There are two other zero-calorie natural sweeteners that we want to mention: stevia and monk fruit. Stevia is a naturally occurring sweetener that has zero calories. It is 200 times sweeter than sugar and is sometimes recommended for people with diabetes who need to limit their sugar intake. However, some studies in animals have shown reduced fertility in subjects who consumed stevia,[5] so it may be best avoided for those trying to conceive. Monk fruit sweetener is derived from part of the monk fruit plant, the mogrosides. It has been used in Traditional Chinese Medicine (TCM) for its anti-inflammatory healing properties. It has zero calories and is about 150 to 250 times sweeter than sugar. People with diabetes may use monk fruit that has not been combined with other sweeteners as an alternative to sugar. Thus far, it appears safe for those who are trying to conceive and want to avoid sugar, but be aware that the high sweetness level may dull your taste buds for the natural sweetness of whole fruit.

So how should we be thinking about sugar, natural sweeteners, and artificial sweeteners when it comes to a fertility-promoting diet? In our Food-First Fertility Plan, we recommend limiting added sugars to less than 5 percent of total daily calories to avoid the glucose spikes and chronic inflammation that can harm your fertility. For most people, this would be about 6 teaspoons, or 25 grams, per day. Whole fruits need not be limited since they have fiber to slow down sugar absorption, as well as a plethora of vitamins, minerals, and antioxidants. In fact, a piece of fruit or a bowl of berries after dinner is a great, naturally sweet dessert that you can enjoy daily.

As you cook more at home, it is fine to use a little real sugar or natural sweeteners such as honey, maple syrup, or date syrup. Sweet is one of our main tastes, after all, and natural sweeteners are used to balance the flavors in some recipes. We know that using sugar and natural sweeteners at home is better for your overall health than buying ultra-processed foods and beverages with added sugars. Keep the super sweet coffee drinks, tea drinks, sodas, sports drinks, and sweet baked goods as less frequent treats rather than everyday occurrences. And take a pass on zero-calorie sweeteners. Remember that nothing needs to be off limits, but added sugars and artificial sweeteners do not offer the nutrient density you are looking for when you are trying to conceive. When an individual consumes too much added sugar or sweeteners, foods that are naturally sweet, like fruit, don't taste sweet enough. Your palate can be retrained, however, by reducing the number of added sugars you consume. Some people need to go cold turkey from store-bought sweets or drinks to reduce the dopamine reward cycle in the brain from high sugar intake. Over a couple of weeks, you should be able to taste the sweetness of fruits again and enjoy them as your daily sweet indulgence.

Alcohol

More than half of adults in the United States drink alcohol on a regular basis. An occasional glass of wine with your partner can complement a romantic dinner, and going out for a drink with friends can encourage bonding and community. But chronic use can lead to harmful mental and physical consequences. When alcohol is metabolized, it turns into acetaldehyde, which is a toxin to tissues in our bodies. It is known to cause inflammation and oxidative stress, which, as we know, can potentially harm sperm, eggs, and the uterine lining. Heavy consumption of alcohol can disrupt the gut microbiota and increase gut permeability and dysbiosis.[6]

Alcohol also increases the risk of breast cancer and other cancers. It has been classified as a group 1 carcinogen by the WHO. As little as one drink per day can increase the risk of hormone receptor positive breast cancer by damaging DNA and temporarily increasing circulating estrogen levels.[7] So, honestly, the health effects of alcohol are pretty one-sided.

For couples undergoing IVF, alcohol consumption immediately before or during the cycle has shown reduced outcomes. One study showed the IVF failure rate to be four times as high for women who drank alcohol one month prior to the IVF cycle compared to those who didn't. Four or more drinks per week reduced the odds of a live birth.[8] Men who drank alcohol one month prior to or during an IVF cycle also had less successful outcomes.[9] In a meta-analysis that combined results from fourteen studies and included about 27,000 people, alcohol consumption of about a glass of wine per day decreased live birth rates for both women and men by 7 and 9 percent, respectively, compared to those who abstained.[10] There has also been a lower birth rate and higher observed miscarriage rate when either men or women drank alcohol immediately before an IVF cycle.[11]

Although not every study has shown a decrease in fertility with light to moderate alcohol consumption, there seems to be a stronger relationship to fertility when it comes to heavier alcohol use. A meta-analysis combing nineteen studies and close to one hundred thousand women pursuing natural conception observed a dose-related decrease in fertility with more alcohol consumption.[12] In other words, alcohol most likely reduces fertility and increases miscarriage in conjunction with consumption, that is, the more alcohol consumed, the more negative the impact.

If you choose to continue to consume alcohol while trying to conceive, the amount and timing may matter. Light to moderate consumption has less of an effect than heavier consumption, and drinking during the first half of the menstrual cycle appears to have less influence than during the second half of the menstrual cycle.[13] If you are putting a large investment of time and money into an IVF cycle, you may want to abstain completely for at least one month prior to and during the IVF cycle to minimize any negative impact on sperm and eggs. Abstaining for two to three months prior to IVF may be even better, but that timespan has not been studied. You should also abstain from alcohol during the month of the embryo transfer and beyond to avoid any effect on implantation and pregnancy.

Most people are aware there is no safe level of alcohol consumption during pregnancy, so full abstinence is recommended. Alcohol is a known teratogen, meaning it causes birth defects. A child who was exposed to alcohol in utero can experience metabolic disorders and neurodevelopmental effects from changes around their DNA, and moderate to heavy alcohol exposure can lead to severe conditions presenting as fetal alcohol spectrum disorder.[14,15]

Smoking

Smoking is the leading cause of morbidity and mortality worldwide. It increases rates of cancer, lung disease, heart disease, and stroke. And yet, about 20 percent of adults in the United States continue to use nicotine and about one billion people smoke worldwide. Tobacco use fell when the increased risk of lung cancer was finally brought to light in 1964 by the U.S. Surgeon General's report, but its use is on the rise again with e-cigarettes and vaping devices. Nicotine is a highly addictive substance leading to dependency.

Smoking can cause many negative changes in reproductive health that are well documented, such as delaying time to pregnancy, reducing egg supply, and impairing sperm function.[16] Active smoking during the three months leading up to an IVF cycle can cut success rates in half.[17] Recognized risks of smoking during pregnancy include preterm delivery, placental abruption, and intrauterine growth restriction.[18] Smoking causes a higher rate of miscarriage, higher rates of bleeding during pregnancy, and lower birth weight in the newborn.

The data on smoking is decisive. Current smokers have lower pregnancy rates and higher miscarriage rates. Trying to conceive is excellent motivation to quit smoking.

Cannabis

Marijuana comes from the cannabis sativa or cannabis indica plant. Cannabis legalization in many states has led to more people using tetrahydrocannabinol (THC) for its psychoactive, relaxing properties via either inhaled or ingested forms. CBD, or cannabidiol, the nonpsychoactive component of cannabis, can be used to reduce anxiety and help with sleep. By most recent estimates, about 10 percent of women and 15 percent of men use some form of cannabis, either THC or CBD, while trying to conceive.

THC has medical applications, perhaps the most useful being to relieve chemotherapy-induced nausea and vomiting and increase appetite in cancer patients.[19,20] Depending on the user's age and frequency of use, THC can lead to impaired brain development and cognitive function, chronic bronchitis, and addiction.[21,22] When inhaling cannabis, additional chemicals may be delivered, similar to tobacco cigarettes. Cannabis, along with these other inhaled chemicals, may increase risk of testicular cancer.[23]

CBD also binds to cannabinoid receptors and has recognized health applications without the negative effects of THC. CBD has been used medically to treat seizure disorder, chronic pain, anxiety, and insomnia. Although THC and CBD have some health benefits, neither should be used during pregnancy. Some women have used THC to relieve nausea in pregnancy, but this is not recommended due to the harm it can cause to the fetus. Cannabis can also increase the risk of preterm birth.[24] In children whose mothers used cannabis during pregnancy, there is a higher rate of neurodevelopmental delay, as well as ongoing cognitive and behavioral abnormalities. These effects can carry on into adulthood.[25]

Given that cannabis has only recently been legalized, there are very few studies that directly assess its impact on human reproduction. However, given its mechanism of action and data from animal studies, the probable effects on human reproduction are not positive.[26,27] For instance, THC may interact with the hypothalamic pituitary ovarian (HPO) axis[28] and may interfere with follicle development and ovulation by disrupting hormone secretion. In bovine eggs, THC can reduce the number of mature eggs and, for those that fertilize, reduce the number that demonstrate normal cleavage.[29] It can cause alterations in the

DNA of the follicle through chemical changes.[30] It can disturb sperm maturation and function and cause epigenetic changes to the sperm DNA expression.[31] THC can also cause erectile dysfunction, which is not a good thing when trying to conceive.[32] In a study of about 400 men in the Seattle, Washington, area, 17 percent of men were using marijuana while trying to conceive. Their semen analysis showed a lower percentage of normal morphology and volume compared to never users.[33] In another study, among a group of healthy young men who were testing for military service in Denmark, smoking marijuana for three months prior to start of service was shown to decrease sperm count by 28 percent.[34]

Data is limited, but thus far, population studies have not shown an observed reduction in pregnancy rates from cannabis use while trying to conceive.[35,36] However, some individuals may be more affected biologically by cannabis than others. In a group of women who had a history of pregnancy loss, current or prior use of cannabis was associated with reduced fecundability (pregnancy rate per cycle) compared to nonusers.[37] In another small study of women who had previously experienced pregnancy loss, women who used cannabis had a 41 percent reduced chance of conceiving compared to those who did not use cannabis.[38]

Given the negative effect of cannabis seen on sperm and follicle development, and the influence on the HPO axis, it is likely that cannabis may reduce fertility for some people trying to conceive. The best advice is to minimize or abstain from use while trying to conceive and avoid completely once pregnant.

Caffeine

Caffeine is the most widely used recreational drug, with more than 80 percent of people in the United States consuming caffeine daily. Caffeine improves focus and alertness by stimulating the central nervous system and increasing neurotransmitter release in the brain. Coffee and tea are rich in antioxidants and polyphenols, offering health benefits. Coffee has been shown to reduce the risk of certain cancers and increase longevity.

However, high levels of caffeine have been linked to miscarriage and possibly infertility. Caffeine is found in coffee, espresso drinks, black and green tea, chocolate, and energy drinks. An average cup of drip coffee has about 100 to 160 milligrams of caffeine. More than 400 milligrams of caffeine per day may cause unwanted side effects such as jitteriness, decreased focus, and insomnia.

The effects of caffeine on male fertility are mixed. Some studies have shown that caffeine intake in men may increase the time to pregnancy for their partners. It may also cause more DNA damage to their sperm. Results, however, are inconsistent.[39] In one study, higher caffeine intake in men was associated with lower IVF success rates for their partners.[40]

The effect of caffeine intake on female fertility has also been inconclusive. Several small studies in the 1990s concluded that caffeine may impair fertility, but more recent studies have not validated this relationship.[41] According to a study published in 2022 that looked at caffeine metabolites and time to pregnancy, there did not seem to be any negative relationship at low to moderate levels of consumption.[42] In another study, researchers looked at the relationship between soda consumption and IVF outcomes. Women who drank more sugar-sweetened beverages had worse IVF outcomes compared to those who did not, but no relationship was observed with caffeine intake and female IVF outcomes.[43] In a cohort study, coffee consumption was examined for Danish couples undergoing IUI or IVF. There was no difference seen in IVF, and a potential benefit was seen for IUI.[44] Finally, a meta-analysis published in 2022 looked at twelve studies of couples undergoing IVF/ICSI and found no detrimental relationship between caffeine consumption and outcomes.[45]

As far as miscarriage, the relationship is more defined. The higher the daily caffeine intake, the higher rates of spontaneous abortion and stillbirth.[46] A notable 20 percent higher rate of miscarriage was seen in women who consumed more than 400 milligrams of caffeine per day.[47]

The takeaway message regarding caffeine is to minimize consumption once pregnant. If you are trying to conceive, it's probably okay to consume one cup of coffee per day. For those who are accustomed to drinking more than that, you may want to look at why your body might be craving caffeine. Perhaps you are not getting enough sleep at night, and you are using caffeine to feel alert. Examine your sleep habits and make sure you are getting enough hours of restful sleep to avoid daytime sleepiness. Perhaps you are not giving your body enough nourishment in the morning, and you are substituting caffeine for food. Make sure you have enough healthy food throughout the day to maintain your energy levels, and don't use caffeine as an energy substitute.

Part 2: Environmental Toxins

Test Your Knowledge
Natural cosmetics are free from health risks.* True/False
Reducing exposure to BPA takes months.** True/False

How much do environmental toxins affect your health and fertility? Quite a bit, it turns out. Researchers have found associations between a number of toxic substances and sperm, eggs, and embryos. Endocrine disrupting chemicals, or EDCs, interrupt the normal functioning of hormones.[48] Is it any surprise that these may be best avoided when trying to conceive? We'll tell you how to minimize your exposure to EDCs like BPA, phthalates, PFAS, and pesticides, as well as other toxins like plastics and air pollution.

BPA

Bisphenols are EDCs that can mimic the action of estrogen when they get into your body through ingestion or via the skin. Bisphenol A (BPA) has been used as an epoxy resin to line food cans and as a thermal heat-resistant coating on paper receipts, where it can be absorbed through your skin. Studies have shown

---

* False. "Natural" is not a regulated term in cosmetics. Check the ingredients list and try to avoid parabens, phthalates, fragrances, and perfumes to reduce your exposure to endocrine disruptors.

** False. BPA has a half-life of about forty-eight hours, so reducing your exposure can have an immediate benefit to your fertility. Avoid heating food in plastic and try to replace cans with boxes or glass jars.

that exposure to BPA can lead to newborn health issues, early puberty, breast cancer, prostate problems, infertility, PCOS, insulin resistance, endometriosis, and miscarriage.[49] The National Toxicology Program of the National Institutes of Health (NIH) officially declared BPA unsafe in 2007. Companies have voluntarily been removing BPA from their food cans, plastic bottles, and baby formula cans. Even now, BPA is not officially banned in the United States, although its use is restricted in many states.

As BPA is pulled off the market in certain areas, it is being replaced by other equally harmful bisphenols like bisphenol S and bisphenol F, which have the same endocrine-disrupting and toxic effects as BPA.[50] This phenomenon, substituting one toxic chemical for another, was described in a *Washington Post* op-ed as "chemical whack-a-mole."[51] Once one chemical is removed and replaced by another, scientists need to spend the time accumulating data to prove that the substitute chemical is equally unsafe before those new chemicals are removed from common use, prolonging our exposure to potentially toxic chemicals. Because all bisphenols may have similar endocrine-disrupting effects, it is best to reduce consumption of canned foods and avoid accepting thermal receipts when possible.

That being said, it is unlikely that we will be able to avoid all bisphenols. Canned beans, lentils, fruits, and vegetables are common pantry items that can be super useful when trying to prepare a quick meal. We keep plenty of cans of food in our pantry when we don't have time for lengthier preparations. And honestly, the benefit of consuming canned beans outweighs the risk of bisphenol exposure, in our opinion. It is much better to eat beans and have a small amount of bisphenol exposure than to not eat beans, just like our recommendation to eat conventionally grown vegetables if they are easier to access or are more affordable than organic varieties. We'd rather see you eat lots of vegetables (after rinsing them off) than worry about any trace amount of residual pesticides. When you pull out a can of beans or vegetables, just rinse them well, too, before consuming, and enjoy! Rinsing canned beans has been shown to reduce the amount of residual BPA.[52] And they have too many nutrients to pass up.

Phthalates

Phthalates (the "ph" is silent) are common EDCs found in household and beauty supplies, including cosmetics, shampoos, soaps, and perfumes, and are used as plasticizers in polyvinyl chloride (PVC). In animal and lab studies, phthalates have been shown to disrupt follicular development and potentially accelerate ovarian aging.[53] They can also affect how sperm DNA is expressed by changing which genes get turned on and off.[54] Phthalates can be tricky to discern and avoid. One of the easiest ways to reduce your exposure to phthalates is to avoid buying anything scented. Try to use the most natural cleaning products or make your own at home. Websites like millionmarker.com can help you locate bisphenols and phthalates in your home and learn how to pick safer products. You can even send in your urine to get a profile of how many toxic chemicals are in your body.

Parabens

Parabens are another EDC typically used as a preservative in cosmetics and personal care products. They are antibacterial and antifungal, thus increasing the shelf life of the products to which they're added. Parabens, along with BPA and triclosan, another chemical preservative, have been associated with infertility.[55] Parabens have been shown to decrease antral follicle counts and increase miscarriage.[56] Reduce your exposure to parabens by reading the labels of your cosmetics and hair-care products and avoiding any that have a paraben ingredient listed (chemicals from parabens end with "-paraben" in the name).

PFAS

Per- and poly-fluorinated alkyl substances (PFAS) are another group of EDCs used as water and stain repellants on clothing, furniture, carpets, outdoor gear, and nonstick skillets. These chemicals contain a very strong carbon-fluorine bond that can resist oil and water and get distributed in our environment over time. They are known as forever chemicals because they have a very long half-life, so their levels just keep accumulating.[57] Some PFAS can cause testicular cancer, kidney cancer, and immune suppression, and interfere with body weight regulation. The health effects of PFAS and forever chemicals are just starting to be observed. It may take some time to discover their direct effects on fertility, but they have been seen in follicular fluid in patients undergoing IVF.[58,59] They appear to be carcinogenic and reduce ovarian reserve, potentially leading to earlier menopause.[60] You can reduce exposure to PFAS by avoiding clothing, furniture, and outdoor gear that has been coated with water or stain repellants. Also, avoid "nonstick" skillets and use safer cookware made of materials like iron, stainless steel, or ceramic.

Microplastics

Plastics are ubiquitous in our food supply and packaging. They make up a huge percentage of the food containers (both in the grocery store and at restaurants) we use, and many of the other household products we buy. These plastics take more than a lifetime to break down. As they start to break down (becoming microplastics), they enter the oceans and our freshwater supply. From there, they enter our bodies. We do not yet know what health risks these microplastics will pose to our health, as they are only now starting to be studied.[61] We also do not know how they will affect fertility or miscarriage risk, but there is already some evidence that they may lower sperm counts in animal models,[62] and potentially in humans.[63] In a mouse model, exposure to microplastics lowered hormone levels and resulted in fewer embryos and lower pregnancy rates.[64] Your best bet to reducing your exposure to the toxic effects of microplastics is to avoid single-use plastic water bottles and avoid heating any type of plastic container in the microwave. You should also avoid putting hot foods into plastic storage containers. Ideally, replace plastic food storage containers with safer alternatives. Stick to glass, paper, or stainless steel when available.

Air Pollution

Air pollution has increased in industrialized cities and travels far and wide. It can be caused by anything from car emissions to factory emissions to wildfires. Fine particulate matter from wildfires can travel thousands of miles.[65] Air pollution that is outside can seep into our homes and places of work, and indoor air pollutants typically register at about half the level of what they are outdoors.[66] Air contaminants increase inflammation and oxidative stress. They have been shown to decrease animal and human fertility by causing defects in gametes and reducing pregnancy rates each month.[67,68] Women exposed to higher levels of air pollution have worse outcomes with IVF treatment and higher miscarriage rates.[69] There is even data suggesting that higher exposure to particulates may accelerate ovarian aging.[70] To protect yourself against air pollution, consider a HEPA air filter in your home and wear a high-quality mask like a KN95 or N95 when particulate matter outside registers as dangerous or high.

Pesticides

Pesticides are yet another class of chemicals that we are inadvertently exposed to in our food supply. A number of studies have shown that sperm demonstrate impairment in function and DNA integrity with higher exposure to pesticides.[71] Even organically grown produce has residual, measurable amounts of pesticides, albeit in smaller amounts than conventionally grown produce. And low levels of pesticides and herbicides like glyphosate are endocrine disruptors and harm female fertility.[72] To reduce pesticide intake, rinse any fruits and vegetables thoroughly with water prior to cooking or eating. You can further minimize pesticide exposure by buying local produce from a farmers market, community-supported agriculture (CSA), or the organic produce section of the grocery store when possible.

Gabriela's Story

Gabriela conceived naturally after about a year of trying. At about eight weeks, she suspected something was wrong. Her husband, Mark, remained hopeful, but an ultrasound confirmed a miscarriage. After the loss and additional months of trying, Gabriela's ob-gyn suggested they seek fertility treatment and consider IVF since they desired more than one child. While they prepared for IVF, they completed two cycles of IUI without success. All their fertility testing turned up normal results.

Gabriela stopped drinking alcohol when they started trying to conceive. They wanted to be sure they were doing everything else they could to optimize their success and scheduled a meeting with Judy. She talked to Gabriela about reducing the red meat and sweet treats in her diet and adding more fish for the omega-3s. Judy also discussed endocrine disruptors in Gabriela's beauty products. She assured Gabriela and Mark that she could guide them to find alternative hair care, skin care, makeup, and cleaning products that would be safer. Gabriela was hesitant about changing the brands that she loved.

At their follow-up session, Gabriela brought multiple bags of self-care products and poured them out on Judy's large office table. They sorted through the dozens of bottles, tubes, and jars, and Mark promised he would help her replace all of them with gentle products without endocrine disruptors. On their way home they stopped at a store that carried natural products without phthalates and bought new fragrance-free alternatives.

It was almost a three-year journey until they received the results that they were pregnant. At her embryo transfer Gabriela felt calm and described a "feeling like a flutter of butterflies inside her." She knew her baby had found their space. Focusing on positive changes in her diet, reducing endocrine disruptors (from all her products), and adding yoga and acupuncture were all so helpful. To this day, she misses her perfumes and fragranced products but shares that it was worth it.

Takeaways

1. Alcohol consumption decreases pregnancy rates and increases miscarriage rates during IVF cycles.
2. Tobacco negatively impacts many aspects of reproductive health. It decreases fertility and increases miscarriage.
3. Cannabis may reduce fertility in some individuals and may increase miscarriage.
4. High caffeine intake may increase miscarriage.
5. All endocrine-disrupting chemicals (EDCs) including BPA, phthalates, PFAS, pesticides, and others may accelerate ovarian aging and decrease male and female fertility.
6. Air pollution may harm fertility.

Sample SMART Goals

1. Look for hidden sugars and artificial sweeteners in foods and beverages and try to avoid them.
2. Cut back or eliminate tobacco, alcohol, and marijuana. Avoid situations and triggers associated with the undesired habit/s.
3. Cut back on caffeine if it is interfering with sleep or if you are pregnant.
4. Minimize consumption of canned foods and exposure to thermal receipts to avoid bisphenols.
5. Minimize hidden phthalates and parabens in household and skincare products. Labels must list ingredients but don't have to specifically disclose that they contain parabens or phthalates. Phthalates can be reduced by avoiding added fragrances. Chemicals from parabens end with "-paraben" in the name. Look for skincare brands that are completely free of EDCs.
6. Avoid plastic containers and cans of food and beverages, and do not microwave or put hot food into plastic containers, even those marked "microwave-safe," because some of the packaging material can migrate into the food when heated. Use glass, stainless steel, or silicone for food storage.

Chapter 13

The Blueprint: Your Six-Week Guide

Test Your Knowledge

Changing my eating habits will be hard.* True/False

Eating a plant-forward diet will help me improve my chance at conception.**
True/False

Finally, we've come to the blueprint! We know that changing your diet can be difficult. That is why we came up with this six-week transition plan, modeled after our class, to help you get started on a fertility-promoting diet. Remember, this plan is for *you* and can be customized depending on your situation and particular goals. It can take as long or short a time as you'd like; you may want to repeat a week and take a little longer at certain points or speed up the schedule as it meets your needs. As you adopt new habits, remember, you'll be making progress, not looking for

---

* True, but it can be done! Setting weekly goals that are realistic for you can form lasting habits. Check out our six-week blueprint for guidance and ask for support from friends and family.

** True! Reading our book, setting goals, and enjoying a plant-forward diet will provide you with nutrition and health to improve your fertility.

perfection. Have grace and acceptance for yourself and the process. We're rooting for you!

The Blueprint

The fertility blueprint is a framework we designed for those of you who would like guidance adopting the Food-First Fertility Plan to gradually change your habits over six weeks. You may be transitioning from an omnivore diet to a flexitarian diet or going toward a vegetarian diet. Regardless of your situation, this blueprint is meant to be personalized and modified as you see fit. It is paced to slowly increase your consumption of vegetables and legumes and build up other health-enhancing habits. Where you are starting from and where you end up are unique for each person. It's not one size fits all.

There are two main reasons to take the dietary transition slowly. First, increasing fiber too quickly in your diet can cause bloating and gas. It would be very uncomfortable to move immediately from 10 grams of fiber per week to 30 grams per week. When you are adding more vegetables and legumes into your diet, you need to give your gut microbiota time to catch up, multiply, and settle into their new routine.

Second, it takes a decent amount of time to change any habit. Changing your diet can be especially challenging as you may be modifying tastes, foods, and traditions that you are accustomed to enjoying. If you try to jump in all at once without first developing the culinary skills to sustain a plant-forward approach, you may feel overwhelmed and give up.

For most individuals, incorporating changes over a six-week period has proven to be a more effective strategy than changing too much at once. Look at modifying your diet as a fun exploration as you broaden the foods you welcome into your meals. Find joy in different cuisines and savor new flavors. This blueprint will help you expand and enhance your home cooking by adding new foods, spices, and recipes each week. A good target is to establish five staple recipes that you love and can cook from memory. Experiment with new plant-forward recipes each week and add them to your staples list when you find a hit. Beyond six weeks, your new fertility-promoting habits will continue to blossom.

As you work your way through the blueprint, remember to use any of your prior weekly SMART goals. Here are some additional ideas to help you get started:

- Plan your meals around the stars: vegetables. They're your *best* antioxidant and fiber friends.
- Enjoy plant-based proteins daily. Beans, lentils, edamame, and peas rank highest.
- If it's a simple carb, combine it with fiber or protein.
- Supercharge one meal each day with a bowl of beautiful greens and a homemade vinaigrette.
- Make a grain bowl instead of a sandwich. You'll be using whole grains instead of processed grains. It's also a perfect place for legumes or a protein flip.
- Visualize changes in your eating habits leading to more motivation and more positive changes, and so on, in an upward spiral.

Week 1

- Watch a knife skills video and practice your cutting skills. Being fast and efficient with food prep will make cooking much more enjoyable.
- Take a prenatal vitamin with folic acid.
- Start each day with a plan for your meals and snacks.

Fruits and Vegetables

- Aim for three servings of fruits and vegetables per day.
- Make a kale or spinach salad recipe (try the Massaged Kale Salad with Citrus and Pomegranate recipe on page 57).
- Eat a serving of berries.

Legumes

- Cook dried white beans, or use a can or box of white beans, rinsing thoroughly.
- Add a base aromatic trio to a legume dish, such as sofrito base from Spain: garlic, onion, and tomato with cooked white beans.

Activate

- Take a relaxing ten-minute walk after dinner to reduce post-meal glucose levels.

Week 2

- Practice being mindful when you eat. Take a few breaths before you start and appreciate the bounty of your meal. How does it taste and feel when you start eating?
- Plan, shop, and prep food on Sunday or another day.

Fruits and Vegetables

- Aim for four servings of fruits and vegetables per day.
- Supercharge one meal each day with a mix of greens and a homemade vinaigrette.
- Add a cruciferous vegetable: try some cauliflower, roasted, steamed, or raw.
- Prep a veggie snack for midweek: carrots and snap peas.

Legumes

- Try lentils!

- Add a base aromatic trio to a legume dish, such as mirepoix from France: onions, carrots, and celery added to French lentils or black beluga lentils.

Activate

- Add a ten-minute wake-up walk in the morning to reset your circadian clock.

Week 3

- Become attuned to your hunger and satiety.
- Continue to increase the variety of your foods.
- Savor the experience of eating a home-cooked meal.
- On Sunday, plan, prep, and batch cook enough beans for two to three meals.

Fruits and Vegetables

- Aim for two servings of fruit and three servings of vegetables per day.
- Have a leafy salad with homemade vinaigrette.
- Have a cruciferous vegetable daily. We love steamed broccoli with garlic and EVOO!
- Try a new local fruit in season.

Legumes

- Pick a type of bean and soak 1 cup overnight. Cook it the next day.
- Add a base aromatic trio to a legume dish, such as this one from West Africa: chili pepper, onions, and tomatoes with black-eyed peas or black beans.

Whole Grains

- Try an ancient grain: farro, quinoa, or wheat berries.

Fish

- Try a fatty fish recipe (such as the Sheet Pan Salmon and Broccoli recipe on page 144).

Activate

- Add a ten-minute walk after lunch every day, and ten minutes of strength training and stretching with yoga or resistance bands twice a week.

Week 4

- Continue to explore movement that brings you pleasure.
- Think about some staple recipes with which you are getting comfortable.
- On Sunday, plan and prep snacks for three days.
- Batch cook some beans or grains.

Fruits and Vegetables

- Aim for six servings per day.
- Continue to enjoy a daily salad with added colorful vegetables and a homemade vinaigrette.
- Try another cruciferous vegetable such as cabbage; stir fry, roast, or sauté to cook. Continue to incorporate at least one per day.
- Add some mushrooms and greens to an egg or tofu scramble.

- Add a red or orange vegetable to a dish: try sweet potato or carrots; steam or roast with garlic or cumin.
- Enjoy some blueberries!
- Make a homemade snack.

Legumes

- Try a soy recipe using tofu, tempeh, or edamame (such as the Stir-Fried Cabbage and Tofu recipe on page 97).
- Add a base aromatic trio to a legume dish, such as this one from New Orleans, Louisiana: onions, green bell pepper, and celery sautéed with tofu or tempeh (optional hot sauce).

Whole Grains

- Try another ancient grain: freekeh, barley, or black rice.

Nuts and Seeds

- Eat a small handful of almonds or other nuts daily for a snack.

Activate

- Go for a green walk: plan a longer weekend hike or a walk through a city park.

Week 5

- Stay attuned to your hunger and fullness. If you feed yourself regularly, you can decide how much you want at each meal.
- On Sunday, plan and prep meals and snacks for three days.
- Repeat a staple meal.

Fruits and Vegetables

- Aim for seven servings of fruits and vegetables per day.
- Include fresh or frozen raspberries with a whole grain porridge or whole-fat yogurt.
- Eat raw or steamed greens every day.
- Cook with alliums: onions, garlic, shallots, or leeks.
- Eat something from the ROY (red, orange, yellow) color families, such as the Sweet Potato Lentil Bowl on page 79.
- Eat cruciferous vegetables most days, steamed, roasted, or stir-fried: broccoli, cauliflower, cabbage, brussels sprouts, or bok choy.

Legumes

- Try a lentil recipe.
- Add a base aromatic trio to a legume dish, such as this one from India: ginger, garlic, and green chilis added to red or green lentils.
- Try a protein flip: add lentils or beans to a dish in place of half the meat.

Whole Grains

- Try another new whole grain: bulgur wheat or millet.
- Make the Quinoa Vegetable Paella recipe on page 59.

Nuts and Seeds

- Add walnuts to full-fat yogurt and whole fruit (see Yogurt Fruit Parfait, page 111).

Activate

- Increase total daily walk time to thirty minutes for a mood boost: ten minutes before breakfast, and ten minutes after lunch and dinner.

Week 6

- Repeat a staple recipe.
- Be adventurous! Try a recipe using new foods or spices.
- On Sunday, plan and prep meals and snacks for three days.
- Batch cook quinoa and use it in two separate dishes this week.

Fruits and Vegetables

- Aim for eight servings of fruits and vegetables per day.
- Keep fresh fruits and vegetables easily available and ready to grab.
- Eat raw or cooked greens every day. Add to scrambles, bowls, and soups.
- Cook with alliums: onions, garlic, shallots, or leeks.
- Eat your daily ROY: make a roasted beet salad. Add chives or parsley.
- Eat cruciferous vegetables most days: broccoli, cauliflower, or brussels sprouts; roast with za'atar, garlic, or paprika.
- Eat your blue, red, and violet fruits; add to any meal.

Legumes

- Eat one to two servings of beans, lentils, or soy most days.
- Add a base aromatic trio to a legume dish, such as this one from Mexico: onions, tomato, and garlic added to black beans or pintos.
- Make a black bean wrap with onion, garlic, tomato, lime, and cilantro.

Nuts and Seeds

- Add toasted pepitas to garnish a dish or salad.

Whole Grains

- Eat at least two servings of whole grains daily. Explore new ancient grains.

Fish

- Try adding small fish like anchovies to a hearty vegetable tomato sauce. Serve over whole grain pasta.

Activate

- Spark joy! Walk ten minutes outdoors in the morning, ten minutes after lunch, and twenty minutes after dinner.

Personalize Your Program

You may choose to obtain personalized advice from a nutrition expert, preferably one specializing in fertility and preconception nutrition. This may be especially important if you have food allergies, sensitivities, or medical conditions that result in reduced intake of certain food groups. Look for the RD (Registered Dietitian) or RDN (Registered Dietitian Nutritionist) title to find individuals with the most training. RDNs are food and nutrition experts with a master's degree from an accredited dietetics program. To hold this title, they must complete a rigorous academic program, work many supervised hours in the field of dietetics, pass a national exam, and complete ongoing professional education throughout their careers.

Nutritionist, as a stand-alone title, is less well defined and can mean different things in different locations. Some nutritionists have gone through a bachelor's degree program or associate degree program, but others have less training, earning a certificate of participation in an online course. Nutritionists, unlike RDNs, are not required to complete a rigorous internship, pass a national exam, or complete continuing education. In some states, nutritionists who have met initial educational requirements will become state licensed or certified. In other states, wearing the nutritionist hat does not require any specific training, testing, licensing, or certification. Make sure to understand if your state certifies or licenses nutritionists and ask about credentials if you choose to see a nutrition expert.

Food-First Fertility Sample Menus

We hope you've had good luck using the blueprint as a template to help incorporate new plant-based foods, spices, and world cuisines into your life to boost your fertility. Your job now is to keep your new habits going. We've included three days of sample menus as an illustration of the Food-First Fertility Plan. The snacks are optional and may be enjoyed mid-morning or mid-afternoon, based on your hunger cues or energy needs. You've already been introduced to some of the recipes in the preceding chapters. Others are so simple that they don't need a recipe. Feel free to adapt any recipe to your liking, or search for variations online.

At the end of each sample day, we counted up the number of servings of fruits and vegetables, legumes, whole grains, nuts, seeds, and fats that made up that day's menu so you can see how all your foods are optimized and meeting the plan goals for your reproductive health. When you think about how the sample meals would fill a fertility plate, you can get a sense that half the meal is fruits and vegetables, about a quarter is whole grains, and a quarter is the plant or animal protein. Most days include some healthy nuts, oils, and occasional dairy. For those who are transitioning from omnivore to flexitarian, a few of the recipes lend themselves to the protein flip or swap. For instance, you could add some ground organic poultry to Lentil Chili (page 130) or add shrimp to a salad or stir fry. The most important thing is that you're making progress, however it works best for you!

Day 1

Breakfast

Garden Frittata (page 129)
Whole wheat toast
Citrus

Lunch

Split Pea Soup (page 95)
Crudité (raw vegetables: carrots, peppers)
Whole grain crackers

Dinner

Massaged Kale Salad with Citrus and Pomegranate (page 57)
Quinoa Vegetable Paella (page 59)
Dark chocolate, 1 ounce

Snacks

Steamed edamame
Fruit and 1 tablespoon nut butter

Day 1 Nutrition Recap

Category	Servings	Foods
Fruits and Vegetables	7 to 9	Onions, shallots, garlic, asparagus, carrots, celery, artichoke hearts, tomatoes, peppers, kale, citrus, pomegranate, apple
Legumes	2 to 3	Chickpeas, split peas, edamame
Nuts and Seeds	1	Walnuts, nut butter
Healthy Fats	1	Extra-virgin olive oil
Whole Grains	2 to 3	Quinoa, whole wheat bread, whole grain crackers

Day 2

Breakfast

Overnight Oats (page 75)
Chopped walnuts
Berries

Lunch

Tuna White Bean Salad (page 146)
Seasonal fruit salad

Dinner

Lentil Chili (page 130)
Whole grain roll
Garden salad with vinaigrette

Snacks

Yogurt Fruit Parfait (page 111)
Celery and hummus

Day 2 Nutrition Recap

Category	Servings	Foods
Fruits and Vegetables	7 to 9	Berries, garlic, lemon, celery, onions, peppers, tomatoes, cilantro, lettuce, apples, oranges
Legumes	2 to 3	White beans, lentils, hummus, soy milk
Nuts and Seeds	1	Walnuts
Healthy Fats	3	Extra-virgin olive oil
Whole Grains	2	Oats, whole grains
Dairy	1	Greek yogurt
Fish	1	Tuna

Day 3

Breakfast

Banana Oat Breakfast Smoothie (page 112)

Lunch

Sweet Potato Lentil Bowl (page 79)
Apple slices

Dinner

Sheet Pan Salmon and Broccoli (page 144)
Farro

Snacks

Pistachio Chia Pudding (page 160)
Blueberries and almonds

Day 3 Nutrition Recap

Category	Servings	Foods
Fruits and Vegetables	7 to 9	Sweet potatoes, beets, kale, garlic, lemon, banana, spinach, broccoli, ginger, lime, blueberries, apple
Legumes	1	Lentils
Nuts and Seeds	2 to 3	Almonds, chia seeds, tahini, nut butter, sesame seeds
Healthy Fats	1 to 2	Extra-virgin olive oil, avocado oil
Whole Grains	2 to 3	Farro, quinoa, oats
Fish	1	Salmon

Final Thoughts

Congratulations! You've reached the end of our program to optimize your health and ready yourself for pregnancy. We hope you have incorporated many changes to enhance your fertility, including moving to a plant-forward diet, exercising regularly, managing stress, and connecting with friends often to help you through your fertility journey. By strengthening your diet and lifestyle, you have lowered inflammation, reduced insulin resistance and oxidative stress, and initiated changes to improve your body's receptivity for embryo creation and implantation. These changes can enhance your mood, build up your resilience, and improve your reproductive health. They will continue to benefit you through pregnancy and beyond. Lowering inflammation will also reduce your future risk of diabetes, heart disease, and cancer. Our wish for you is to achieve your best health while you are trying to conceive.

As you move on with your fertility journey, we wish you all the best success. Remember that eating to optimize your fertility is not a diet, and the foods you choose to eat will be different from someone across the street or in another part of the world. The principles of eating well to optimize your health follow certain principles. Once you have completed the six-week blueprint program, and you're feeling strong, continue to follow the guidelines and keep it going, especially through pregnancy and beyond. When you are planning your meals or eating out, ask yourself these questions:

1. Does it have fiber (anti-inflammatory)?
2. Is it low glycemic?
3. Does it contain antioxidants?

Most whole foods from plants are going to check all three of these boxes and be fertility promoters. These three qualities are the most important, big-picture components of a fertility-promoting diet, but, as we've learned, there are some other helpful guidelines to keep in mind if you want to optimize your fertility and overall health. Here are our top ten:

Getting to Baby *Top Ten Tips*

1. Eat the rainbow! Get eight servings of fruits and vegetables (antioxidants and fiber) daily.
2. Fiber city! Eat beans or lentils (protein and fiber) most days.
3. Embrace soy. Eat tofu, tempeh, or edamame (protein and fiber) two to three times per week.
4. Go fish! Eat two to three servings of fatty fish or seafood (protein and antioxidants) per week.
5. Get nutty. Eat a handful of nuts or seeds (antioxidants and fiber) every day.
6. Spice it up. Keep your palate engaged with a world of spices (antioxidants).
7. Discover ancient grains. Eat ancient whole grains (fiber) every day.
8. Cook with EVOO. Use extra-virgin olive oil or avocado oil (anti-inflammatory, antioxidant) for a source of healthy fat.
9. Keep it simple. Drink filtered tap water (nothing added!).
10. Boost it! Walk for ten minutes in the morning, ten minutes after lunch, and twenty minutes after dinner (lowers glycemic effect of foods, anti-inflammatory).

The fertility disruptors are just as important as the fertility promoters. If you can avoid some of the factors that can damage sperm and eggs in the first place, you'll be ahead of the curve. It's best to minimize or avoid things that contribute to inflammation, glycemic spikes, insulin resistance, and oxidative stress.

How to Minimize Fertility Disruptors

1. Not your friends: ultra-processed foods; processed, enriched, fortified grains (high glycemic, low fiber, inflammatory).
2. Steer clear: excess sugars and artificial sweeteners (high glycemic, low fiber, inflammatory).
3. Move to the back of the line: red meat and processed meats (no fiber, inflammatory).
4. Run from the fryer: deep-fried foods (inflammatory, high in omega-6s).
5. Avoid substances: tobacco, alcohol, cannabis (causes damage to eggs and sperm).
6. Reduce exposure to toxins: bisphenols, phthalates, PFAS, microplastics, air pollution, and pesticides (causes damage to hormones, eggs, and sperm).

You're a Food-First Fertility pro now, and you've graduated with honors! We've shared our top tips and quick lists. You've mastered culinary skills and have accomplished SMART goals along the way. You've acquired knowledge and can gleefully share recipes and flavorful meals with friends. You know what to add to your diet and what to leave behind. You know how to slow down and eat mindfully, give your body what it needs, and enjoy playing with new flavors and foods.

We're so excited for you to cook more and enhance your fertility in your own kitchen! Your motivation and confidence will keep you on track. May your path to parenthood be delicious, joyful, and plant-forward!

Resources

Recipe Resources

California Avocados
www.californiaavocado.com

Culinary Institute of America Plant-Forward Kitchen
www.plantforwardkitchen.org/recipes

Food Network Plant-Based Recipes
www.foodnetwork.com/recipes/photos/plant-based-recipes

Lentils
www.lentils.org

Oldways Preservation Trust
https://oldwayspt.org/recipes

Snap-Ed Live Well Recipes
https://wasnap-ed.org/live-well/recipes/

USA Pulses Recipes
https://pulses.org/us/pulse-recipes/

The Vegetarian Resource Group
www.vrg.org

Whole Grain Council Recipes
https://wholegrainscouncil.org/recipes

Washington State University Farm to Families Produce Recipes
https://extension.wsu.edu/skagit/farm-to-families-recipes-and-local
-food-map/

Fertility Education Resources

American Society for Reproductive Medicine: ReproductiveFacts.org
www.reproductivefacts.org

National Institutes of Health: Eunice Kennedy Shriver National Institute of Child Health and Human Development
www.nichd.nih.gov/health/topics/infertility

Resolve: The National Infertility Association
resolve.org

Society for Assisted Reproductive Technology
SART.org

Acknowledgments

The basis for *Getting to Baby* was the Food for Fertility program. Running it was no small task, and many hands helped us along the way. We were supported by several wonderful colleagues at Seattle Reproductive Medicine (SRM) including Marcie Guthrie, who helped with marketing; Jay Yoo and Rori de Leon, who provided technical support when we converted to an online platform; and many at SRM who made sure the kitchen would be clean for our Saturday morning classes. We had a number of graduate students and volunteers who helped with the classes over the years, including Carrie Dennett, Andrea Lopriore, Leah Egbers, Chelsea Hemmenway, Jeani Hunt Gibbons, Francesca Simonella, Srilekha (Lekha) Karunanithi, Kendall (Samford) Altig, and Mary Heid.

Once we started writing *Getting to Baby*, many colleagues from SRM were excited to provide input and try recipes, including the medical assistants, clinic and operating room (OR) nurses, clinical assistants, sonographers, embryologists, and advanced practice providers, among others. I'd like to give a special shout-out to Beth Johnson, who took my chicken challenge seriously and went on a quest to find pasture-raised chicken locally! Thank you to Sarah de la Torre, MD, and the Wellness Team, who always promoted good nutrition and whole health for the patients at SRM. A thank-you also goes out to all of our physician friends at SRM who supported the Food for Fertility classes and supported us writing the book: Nancy Klein, MD; Paul Lin, MD; Amy Criniti,

MD; Lynn Davis, MD, MS; Brenda Houmard, MD, PhD; Gerard Letterie, DO; Nichole Barker, DO; Michele Cho, MD; Erik Mazur, MD; Akhil Shah, MD; and Kaitlyn Wald, MD. Special thanks to Amy, Lynn, and Paul, who've always been incredibly encouraging and supportive.

Other friends who supported us along the way include Mark Ostrow, who helped Angela edit the original proposal while we were on a group vacation to Manzanita, and Becky Benfield, who gave Angela advice on an early draft. Friends Amy Perera and Leisa Goldberg gave valuable feedback on the protein flip and swap chapter, and Diane Ellis, MD, Angela's friend from residency at Oregon Health & Science University (OHSU), gave us great advice on the first few chapters and let us know when the writing was getting a bit too technical.

We'd like to thank our agent, Liz Kracht at Kimberly Cameron & Associates, who took a chance on us after hearing Angela describe the class and the idea for the book at a writers' conference back in 2019. Liz immediately sensed how much a book like this could help women after seeing many of her friends struggle to conceive. Rachel Phares at BenBella has been instrumental in helping to shape the book and hone the writing. Leah Wilson has been an invaluable resource to us. Not only is she an amazing editor, but she's been patient and kind on our journey. She's given exceptional feedback, sharpening the words to keep everything simple and meaningful. We'd like to thank the rest of the team at BenBella as well. They've made the process easy and fun.

Angela is forever grateful to Ben, Ellie, and Kaia, who provided never-ending love and support. Judy is grateful for the unconditional support from Jeff, Elana, Zach, and her mother, Lila. We're both grateful to the wonderful friends and colleagues who've been there to encourage us.

And most of all, thanks to the amazing women who participated in our classes and inspired us to write this book!

Endnotes

Chapter 1 References

1. Dunaif A, Wu X, Lee A, Diamanti-Kandarakis E. Defects in insulin receptor signaling in vivo in the polycystic ovary syndrome (PCOS). Am J Physiol Endocrinol Metab. 2001 Aug;281(2):E392–9. doi: 10.1152/ajpendo.2001.281.2.E392. PMID: 11440917.

2. Crosignani PG, Colombo M, Vegetti W, Somigliana E, Gessati A, Ragni G. Overweight and obese anovulatory patients with polycystic ovaries: Parallel improvements in anthropometric indices, ovarian physiology and fertility rate induced by diet. Hum Reprod. 2003 Sep;18(9):1928–32. doi: 10.1093/humrep/deg367. PMID: 12923151.

3. Practice Committee of the American Society for Reproductive Medicine. Electronic addressasrm@ asrm.org; Practice Committee of the American Society for Reproductive Medicine. Obesity and reproduction: a committee opinion. Fertil Steril. 2021 Nov;116(5):1266–1285. doi: 10.1016/j.fertnstert .2021.08.018. Epub 2021 Sep 25. PMID: 34583840.

4. Basuino L, Silveira CF Jr. Human follicular fluid and effects on reproduction. JBRA Assist Reprod. 2016 Mar 1;20(1):38–40. doi: 10.5935/1518-0557.20160009. PMID: 27203305.

5. Al-Gubory KH. Environmental pollutants and lifestyle factors induce oxidative stress and poor prenatal development. Reprod Biomed Online. 2014 Jul;29(1):17–31. doi: 10.1016/j.rbmo .2014.03.002. Epub 2014 Mar 21. PMID: 24813750.

6. Saben JL, Boudoures AL, Asghar Z, Thompson A, Drury A, Zhang W, Chi M, Cusumano A, Scheaffer S, Moley KH. Maternal metabolic syndrome programs mitochondrial dysfunction via germline changes across three generations. Cell Rep. 2016 Jun 28;16(1):1–8. doi: 10.1016/j.celrep .2016.05.065. Epub 2016 Jun 16. PMID: 27320925; PMCID: PMC4957639.

7. Ibid.

8. Patel C, Ghanim H, Ravishankar S, Sia CL, Viswanathan P, Mohanty P, Dandona P. Prolonged reactive oxygen species generation and nuclear factor-kappaB activation after a high-fat, high-carbohydrate meal in the obese. J Clin Endocrinol Metab. 2007 Nov;92(11):4476–4479. doi: 10.1210/jc.2007-0778. Epub 2007 Sep 4. PMID: 17785362.

9. Wang S, Zheng Y, Li J, Yu Y, Zhang W, Song M, Liu Z, Min Z, Hu H, Jing Y, He X, Sun L, Ma L, Esteban CR, Chan P, Qiao J, Zhou Q, Izpisua Belmonte JC, Qu J, Tang F, Liu GH. Single-cell transcriptomic atlas of primate ovarian aging. Cell. 2020 Feb 6;180(3):585–600.e19. doi: 10.1016/j .cell.2020.01.009. Epub 2020 Jan 30. PMID: 32004457.

10. Wang L, Tang J, Wang L, Tan F, Song H, Zhou J, Li F. Oxidative stress in oocyte aging and female reproduction. J Cell Physiol. 2021 Dec;236(12):7966–7983. doi: 10.1002/jcp.30468. Epub 2021 Jun 14. PMID: 34121193.

11. Chiu YH, Chavarro JE, Souter I. Diet and female fertility: doctor, what should I eat? Fertil Steril. 2018 Sep;110(4):560–569. doi: 10.1016/j.fertnstert.2018.05.027.

12. Chavarro JE, Rich-Edwards JW, Rosner BA, Willett WC. Diet and lifestyle in the prevention of ovulatory disorder infertility. Obstet Gynecol. 2007 Nov;110(5):1050–8. doi: 10.1097/01.AOG .0000287293.25465.e1. PMID: 17978119.

13. Jorge E. Chavarro MD, ScD and Walter C. Willett, MD, DrPH. *The Fertility Diet: Groundbreaking Research Reveals Natural Ways to Boost Ovulation and Improve Your Chances of Getting Pregnant.* New York, NY: McGraw-Hill, 2008.

14. Toledo E, Lopez-del Burgo C, Ruiz-Zambrana A, et al. Dietary patterns and difficulty conceiving: a nested case-control study. Fertility and sterility. 2011; 96:1149–1153. doi: 10.1016/fertnster .2011.08.034.

15. Vujkovic M, de Vries JH, Lindemans J, Macklon NS, van der Spek PJ, Steegers EA, Steegers-Theunissen RP. The preconception Mediterranean dietary pattern in couples undergoing in vitro fertilization/intracytoplasmic sperm injection treatment increases the chance of pregnancy. Fertil Steril. 2010 Nov;94(6):2096–2101. doi: 10.1016/j.fertnstert.2009.12.079. Epub 2010 Mar 1. PMID: 20189169.

16. Twigt JM, Bolhuis ME, Steegers EA, Hammiche F, van Inzen WG, Laven JS, Steegers-Theunissen RP. The preconception diet is associated with the chance of ongoing pregnancy in women undergoing IVF/ICSI treatment. Hum Reprod. 2012 Aug;27(8):2526–2531. doi: 10.1093/humrep/des157. Epub 2012 May 15. PMID: 22593431.

17. Salas-Huetos A, Bulló M, Salas-Salvadó J. Dietary patterns, foods and nutrients in male fertility parameters and fecundability: a systematic review of observational studies. Hum Reprod Update. 2017 Jul 1;23(4):371–389. doi: 10.1093/humupd/dmx006. PMID: 28333357.

18. Gaskins AJ, Nassan FL, Chiu YH, Arvizu M, Williams PL, Keller MG, Souter I, Hauser R, Chavarro JE; EARTH Study Team. Dietary patterns and outcomes of assisted reproduction. Am J Obstet Gynecol. 2019 Jun;220(6):567.e1–567.e18. doi: 10.1016/j.ajog.2019.02.004. Epub 2019 Feb 8. PMID: 30742825; PMCID: PMC6545142.

19. Elkafas H, Wall M, Al-Hendy A, Ismail N. Gut and genital tract microbiomes: dysbiosis and link to gynecological disorders. Front Cell Infect Microbiol. 2022 Dec 16;12:1059825. doi: 10.3389 /fcimb.2022.1059825. PMID: 36590579; PMCID: PMC9800796.

20. Baker JM, Al-Nakkash L, Herbst-Kralovetz MM. Estrogen-gut microbiome axis: physiological and clinical implications. Maturitas. 2017 Sep;103:45–53. doi: 10.1016/j.maturitas.2017.06.025. Epub 2017 Jun 23. PMID: 28778332.

21. Qi X, Yun C, Pang Y, Qiao J. The impact of the gut microbiota on the reproductive and metabolic endocrine system. Gut Microbes. 2021 Jan-Dec;13(1):1–21. doi: 10.1080/19490976.2021.1894070. PMID: 33722164; PMCID: PMC7971312.

22. Yurtdaş G, Akdevelioğlu Y. A New Approach to Polycystic Ovary Syndrome: The Gut Microbiota. J Am Coll Nutr. 2020 May–Jun;39(4):371–382. doi: 10.1080/07315724.2019.1657515. Epub 2019 Sep 12. PMID: 31513473.

23. Ibid.

24. Szendroedi J, Phielix E, Roden M. The role of mitochondria in insulin resistance and type 2 diabetes mellitus. Nat Rev Endocrinol. 2011 Sep 13;8(2):92–103. doi: 10.1038/nrendo.2011.138. PMID: 21912398.

25. Hurrle S, Hsu WH. The etiology of oxidative stress in insulin resistance. Biomed J. 2017 Oct;40(5):257–262. doi: 10.1016/j.bj.2017.06.007. Epub 2017 Nov 8. PMID: 29179880; PMCID: PMC6138814.

26. Henriksen EJ, Diamond-Stanic MK, Marchionne EM. Oxidative stress and the etiology of insulin resistance and type 2 diabetes. Free Radic Biol Med. 2011 Sep 1;51(5):993–999. doi: 10.1016/j.freeradbiomed.2010.12.005. Epub 2010 Dec 13. PMID: 21163347; PMCID: PMC3071882.

27. Wang S, Zheng Y, Li J, Yu Y, Zhang W, Song M, Liu Z, Min Z, Hu H, Jing Y, He X, Sun L, Ma L, Esteban CR, Chan P, Qiao J, Zhou Q, Izpisua Belmonte JC, Qu J, Tang F, Liu GH. Single-cell transcriptomic atlas of primate ovarian aging. Cell. 2020 Feb 6;180(3):585–600.e19. doi: 10.1016/j.cell.2020.01.009. Epub 2020 Jan 30. PMID: 32004457.

28. Chiu YH, Chavarro JE, Souter I. Diet and female fertility: doctor, what should I eat? Fertil Steril. 2018 Sep;110(4):560–569. doi: 10.1016/j.fertnstert.2018.05.027. PMID: 30196938.

29. Showell MG, Mackenzie-Proctor R, Jordan V, Hart RJ. Antioxidants for female subfertility. Cochrane Database Syst Rev. 2020 Aug 27;8(8):CD007807. doi: 10.1002/14651858.CD007807.pub4. PMID: 32851663; PMCID: PMC8094745.

30. Budani MC, Tiboni GM. Effects of supplementation with natural antioxidants on oocytes and pre-implantation embryos. Antioxidants (Basel). 2020 Jul 12;9(7):612. doi: 10.3390/antiox9070612. PMID: 32664650; PMCID: PMC7402117.

31. de Ligny W, Smits RM, Mackenzie-Proctor R, Jordan V, Fleischer K, de Bruin JP, Showell MG. Antioxidants for male subfertility. Cochrane Database Syst Rev. 2022 May 4;5(5):CD007411. doi: 10.1002/14651858.CD007411.pub5. PMID: 35506389; PMCID: PMC9066298.

Chapter 2 References

1. Satter, Ellyn. *Secrets of Feeding a Healthy Family: How to Eat, How to Raise Good Eaters, How to Cook.* Kelcy Press, 2008.

2. Tribole, Evelyn, and Resch, Elyse. *Intuitive Eating.* New York: St. Martin's Griffin, 4th edition, 2020.

3. Habibi N, Hall KA, Moran LJ, Haag DG, Hodge AM, Grieger JA. Is the association between age and fertility problems modified by diet quality? Findings from a national study of reproductive

age women in australia. Nutrients. 2022 Oct 18;14(20):4355. doi: 10.3390/nu14204355. PMID: 36297039; PMCID: PMC9606952.

4. www.sart.org.

Chapter 3 References

1. Watzl B. Anti-inflammatory effects of plant-based foods and of their constituents. Int J Vitam Nutr Res. 2008 Dec;78(6):293–298. doi: 10.1024/0300-9831.78.6.293. PMID: 19685439.

2. Godman, Heidi. How many fruits and vegetables do we really need? Harvard Health Letter, September 1, 2021. www.health.hardvard.edu/nutrition/how-many-fruits-and-vegetables-do-we-really-need.

3. What we eat in America, NHANES, 2007–2010, Dietary Guidelines for Americans, 2015–2020, Health.gov.

4. U.S. Department of Health and Human Services, U.S. Department of Agriculture. *2015–2020 Dietary Guidelines for American*: Washington, DC; 2015. (Dietary Guidelines Advisory Committee. 2020. *Scientific Report of the 2020 Dietary Guidelines Advisory Committee: Advisory Report to the Secretary of Agriculture and the Secretary of Health and Human Services.* U.S. Department of Agriculture, Agricultural Research Service, Washington, DC. Available at: https://doi.org/10.52570/DGAC2020.)

5. Aune D, Giovannucci E, Boffetta P, Fadnes LT, Keum N, Norat T, Greenwood DC, Riboli E, Vatten LJ, Tonstad S. Fruit and vegetable intake and the risk of cardiovascular disease, total cancer and all-cause mortality: a systematic review and dose-response meta-analysis of prospective studies. Int J Epidemiol. 2017 Jun 1;46(3):1029–1056. doi: 10.1093/ije/dyw319. PMID: 28338764; PMCID: PMC5837313.

6. Oyebode O, Gordon-Dseagu V, Walker A, Mindell JS. Fruit and vegetable consumption and all-cause, cancer and CVD mortality: Analysis of Health Survey for England data. J Epidemiol Community Health. 2014 Sep;68(9):856–862. doi: 10.1136/jech-2013-203500. Epub 2014 Mar 31. PMID: 24687909; PMCID: PMC4145465.

7. Blanchflower, David G., Oswald, Andrew J., and Stewart-Brown, Sarah. Is psychological well-being linked to the consumption of fruit and vegetables? (October 2012). NBER Working Paper No. w18469, Available at SSRN: https://ssrn.com/abstract=2164593.

8. Oyebode O, Gordon-Dseagu V, Walker A, Mindell JS. Fruit and vegetable consumption and all-cause, cancer and CVD mortality: analysis of Health Survey for England data. J Epidemiol Community Health. 2014 Sep;68(9):856–862. doi: 10.1136/jech-2013-203500. Epub 2014 Mar 31. PMID: 24687909; PMCID: PMC4145465.

9. McMartin SE, Jacka FN, Colman I. The association between fruit and vegetable consumption and mental health disorders: evidence from five waves of a national survey of Canadians. Prev Med. 2013 Mar;56(3–4):225–230. doi: 10.1016/j.ypmed.2012.12.016. Epub 2013 Jan 4. PMID: 23295173.

10. Mujcic R, J Oswald A. Evolution of well-being and happiness after increases in consumption of fruit and vegetables. Am J Public Health. 2016 Aug;106(8):1504–10. doi: 10.2105/AJPH.2016.303260. PMID: 27400354; PMCID: PMC4940663.

11. Nguyen-Powanda P, Robaire B. Oxidative stress and reproductive function in the aging male. Biology (Basel). 2020 Sep 11;9(9):282. doi: 10.3390/biology9090282. PMID: 32932761; PMCID: PMC7564187.

12. Wang L, Tang J, Wang L, Tan F, Song H, Zhou J, Li F. Oxidative stress in oocyte aging and female reproduction. J Cell Physiol. 2021 Dec;236(12):7966–7983. doi: 10.1002/jcp.30468. Epub 2021 Jun 14. PMID: 341211930.

13. Ahmed TA, Ahmed SM, El-Gammal Z, Shouman S, Ahmed A, Mansour R, El-Badri N. Oocyte aging: The role of cellular and environmental factors and impact on female fertility. Adv Exp Med Biol. 2020;1247:109–123. doi: 10.1007/5584_2019_456. PMID: 31802446.

14. Gaskins AJ, Chavarro JE. Diet and fertility: a review. Am J Obstet Gynecol. 2018 Apr;218(4):379–389. doi: 10.1016/j.ajog.2017.08.010. Epub 2017 Aug 24. PMID: 28844822; PMCID: PMC5826784.

15. Grieger JA, Grzeskowiak LE, Bianco-Miotto T, Jankovic-Karasoulos T, Moran LJ, Wilson RL, Leemaqz SY, Poston L, McCowan L, Kenny LC, Myers J, Walker JJ, Norman RJ, Dekker GA, Roberts CT. Pre-pregnancy fast food and fruit intake is associated with time to pregnancy. Hum Reprod. 2018 Jun 1;33(6):1063–1070. doi: 10.1093/humrep/dey079. PMID: 29733398.

16. Braga DP, Halpern G, Setti AS, Figueira RC, Iaconelli A Jr., Borges E Jr. The impact of food intake and social habits on embryo quality and the likelihood of blastocyst formation. Reprod Biomed Online. 2015 Jul;31(1):30–38. doi: 10.1016/j.rbmo.2015.03.007. Epub 2015 Mar 27. PMID: 25982093.

17. Chung Y, Melo P, Pickering O, Dhillon-Smith R, Coomarasamy A, Devall A. The association between dietary patterns and risk of miscarriage: a systematic review and meta-analysis. Fertil Steril. 2023 Apr 13:S0015–0282(23)00296-0. doi: 10.1016/j.fertnstert.2023.04.011. Epub ahead of print. PMID: 37061157.

18. Makarem N, Chau K, Miller EC, Gyamfi-Bannerman C, Tous I, Booker W, Catov JM, Haas DM, Grobman WA, Levine LD, McNeil R, Bairey Merz CN, Reddy U, Wapner RJ, Wong MS, Bello NA. Association of a Mediterranean diet pattern with adverse pregnancy outcomes among US women. JAMA Netw Open. 2022 Dec 1;5(12):e2248165. doi: 10.1001/jamanetworkopen .2022.48165. PMID: 36547978.11.

19. Practice bulletin no. 187: Neural tube defects. Obstet Gynecol. 2017 Dec;130(6):e279–e290. doi: 10.1097/AOG.0000000000002412. PMID: 29189693.

20. Fielding JM, Rowley KG, Cooper P, O' Dea K. Increases in plasma lycopene concentration after consumption of tomatoes cooked with olive oil. Asia Pac J Clin Nutr. 2005;14(2):131–136. PMID: 15927929.

21. Liu J, Zhou H, Song L, Yang Z, Qiu M, Wang J, Shi S. Anthocyanins: Promising natural products with diverse pharmacological activities. Molecules. 2021 Jun 22;26(13):3807. doi: 10.3390/molecules 26133807. PMID: 34206588; PMCID: PMC8270296.

22. Panche AN, Diwan AD, Chandra SR. Flavonoids: an overview. J Nutr Sci. 2016 Dec 29;5:e47. doi: 10.1017/jns.2016.41. PMID: 28620474; PMCID: PMC5465813.

23. Chiang C, Mahalingam S, Flaws JA. Environmental contaminants affecting fertility and somatic health. Semin Reprod Med. 2017 May;35(3):241–249. doi: 10.1055/s-0037-1603569. Epub 2017 Jun 28. PMID: 28658707; PMCID: PMC6425478.

24. Dosz EB, Jeffery EH. Modifying the processing and handling of frozen broccoli for increased sulforaphane formation. J Food Sci. 2013 Sep;78(9):H1459–463. doi: 10.1111/1750-3841.12221.

25. How to get 8 daily servings of fruits and vegetables. Performance Triad (P3), June 1, 2023. https://p3.amedd.army.mil/news/how-to/make-healthy-eating-easy/how-to-get-8-daily-servings-of-fruits-and-vegetables.

26. 1-2-3 approach to eating fruits and veggies. Speaking of Health. Mayo Clinic Health System, December 30, 2022. www.mayoclinichealthsystem.org/hometown-health/speaking-of-health/123-approach-to-eating-fruits-and-vegetables.

Chapter 4 References

1. McKeown NM, Meigs JB, Liu S, Saltzman E, Wilson PW, Jacques PF. Carbohydrate nutrition, insulin resistance, and the prevalence of the metabolic syndrome in the Framingham Offspring Cohort. Diabetes Care. 2004 Feb;27(2):538–46. doi: 10.2337/diacare.27.2.538. PMID: 14747241.

2. Gaskins AJ, Chavarro JE. Diet and fertility: a review. Am J Obstet Gynecol. 2018 Apr;218(4):379–389. doi: 10.1016/j.ajog.2017.08.010. Epub 2017 Aug 24. PMID: 28844822; PMCID: PMC5826784.

3. Gaskins AJ, Chiu YH, Williams PL, Keller MG, Toth TL, Hauser R, Chavarro JE; EARTH Study Team. Maternal whole grain intake and outcomes of in vitro fertilization. Fertil Steril. 2016 Jun;105(6):1503–1510.e4. doi: 10.1016/j.fertnstert.2016.02.015. Epub 2016 Feb 28. PMID: 26926253; PMCID: PMC4894002.

4. Gupta S, Hawk T, Aggarwal A, Drewnowski A. Characterizing ultra-processed foods by energy density, nutrient density, and cost. Front Nutr. 2019 May 28;6:70. doi: 10.3389/fnut.2019.00070. PMID: 31231655; PMCID: PMC6558394.

5. Crimarco A, Landry MJ, Gardner CD. Ultra-processed Foods, Weight Gain, and Co-morbidity Risk. Curr Obes Rep. 2022 Sep;11(3):80–92. doi: 10.1007/s13679-021-00460-y. Epub 2021 Oct 22. PMID: 34677812; PMCID: PMC8532572.

Chapter 5 References

1. Dahl WJ, Foster LM, Tyler RT. Review of the health benefits of peas (Pisum sativum L.). Br J Nutr. 2012 Aug;108 Suppl 1:S3–10. doi: 10.1017/S0007114512000852. PMID: 22916813.

2. Polak R, Phillips EM, Campbell A. Legumes: Health benefits and culinary approaches to increase intake. Clin Diabetes. 2015 Oct;33(4):198–205. doi: 10.2337/diaclin.33.4.198. PMID: 26487796; PMCID: PMC4608274.

3. Wang K, Zhao Y, Nie J, Xu H, Yu C, Wang S. Higher HEI-2015 score is associated with reduced risk of depression: Result from NHANES 2005-2016. Nutrients. 2021 Jan 25;13(2):348. doi: 10.3390/nu13020348. PMID: 33503826; PMCID: PMC7911826.

4. Jenkins DJA, Kendall CW, Augustin LS, Mitchell S, Sahye-Pudaruth S, Blanco Mejia S, Chiavaroli L, Mirrahimi A, Ireland C, Bashyam B, Vidgen E, de Souza RJ, Sievenpiper JL, Coveney J, Leiter LA, Josse RG. Effect of legumes as part of a low glycemic index diet on glycemic control and cardiovascular risk factors in type 2 diabetes mellitus: a randomized controlled trial. Arch Intern Med. 2012 Nov 26;172(21):1653–1660. doi: 10.1001/2013.jamainternmed.70. PMID: 23089999.

5. Mullins AP, Arjmandi BH. Health benefits of plant-based nutrition: Focus on beans in cardiometabolic diseases. Nutrients. 2021 Feb 5;13(2):519. doi: 10.3390/nu13020519. PMID: 33562498; PMCID: PMC7915747.

6. Kim SJ, de Souza RJ, Choo VL, Ha V, Cozma AI, Chiavaroli L, Mirrahimi A, Blanco Mejia S, Di Buono M, Bernstein AM, Leiter LA, Kris-Etherton PM, Vuksan V, Beyene J, Kendall CW, Jenkins DJ, Sievenpiper JL. Effects of dietary pulse consumption on body weight: a systematic review and meta-analysis of randomized controlled trials. Am J Clin Nutr. 2016 May;103(5):1213–1223. doi: 10.3945/ajcn.115.124677. Epub 2016 Mar 30. PMID: 27030531.

7. Zhang FF, Haslam DE, Terry MB, Knight JA, Andrulis IL, Daly MB, Buys SS, John EM. Dietary isoflavone intake and all-cause mortality in breast cancer survivors: The Breast Cancer Family Registry. Cancer. 2017 Jun 1;123(11):2070–2079. doi: 10.1002/cncr.30615. Epub 2017 Mar 6. PMID: 28263368; PMCID: PMC5444962.

8. Nechuta SJ, Caan BJ, Chen WY, Lu W, Chen Z, Kwan ML, Flatt SW, Zheng Y, Zheng W, Pierce JP, Shu XO. Soy food intake after diagnosis of breast cancer and survival: an in-depth analysis of combined evidence from cohort studies of US and Chinese women. Am J Clin Nutr. 2012 Jul;96(1):123–32. doi: 10.3945/ajcn.112.035972. Epub 2012 May 30. PMID: 22648714; PMCID: PMC3374736.

9. Didinger C, Thompson HJ. Defining nutritional and functional niches of legumes: A call for clarity to distinguish a future role for pulses in the dietary guidelines for Americans. Nutrients. 2021;13(4):1100. Published 2021 Mar 27. doi:10.3390/nu13041100.

10. Didinger C, Thompson HJ. Defining nutritional and functional niches of legumes: A call for clarity to distinguish a future role for pulses in the dietary guidelines for Americans. Nutrients. 2021;13(4):1100. Published 2021 Mar 27. doi:10.3390/nu13041100.

11. Gaskins AJ, Chavarro JE. Diet and fertility: a review. Am J Obstet Gynecol. 2018 Apr;218(4):379–389. doi: 10.1016/j.ajog.2017.08.010. Epub 2017 Aug 24. PMID: 28844822; PMCID: PMC5826784.

12. Mumford SL, Sundaram R, Schisterman EF, Sweeney AM, Barr DB, Rybak ME, Maisog JM, Parker DL, Pfeiffer CM, Louis GM. Higher urinary lignan concentrations in women but not men are positively associated with shorter time to pregnancy. J Nutr. 2014 Mar;144(3):352–358. doi: 10.3945/jn.113.184820. Epub 2014 Jan 8. PMID: 24401816; PMCID: PMC3927547.

13. Unfer V, Casini ML, Gerli S, Costabile L, Mignosa M, Di Renzo GC. Phytoestrogens may improve the pregnancy rate in in vitro fertilization-embryo transfer cycles: a prospective, controlled, randomized trial. Fertil Steril. 2004 Dec;82(6):1509–1513. doi: 10.1016/j.fertnstert.2004.07.934. PMID: 15589851.

14. Gaskins AJ, Nassan FL, Chiu YH, Arvizu M, Williams PL, Keller MG, Souter I, Hauser R, Chavarro JE; EARTH Study Team. Dietary patterns and outcomes of assisted reproduction. Am J Obstet Gynecol. 2019 Jun;220(6):567.e1–567.e18. doi: 10.1016/j.ajog.2019.02.004. Epub 2019 Feb 8. PMID: 30742825; PMCID: PMC6545142.

15. Mumford SL, Sundaram R, Schisterman EF, Sweeney AM, Barr DB, Rybak ME, Maisog JM, Parker DL, Pfeiffer CM, Louis GM. Higher urinary lignan concentrations in women but not men are positively associated with shorter time to pregnancy. J Nutr. 2014 Mar;144(3):352–358. doi: 10.3945/jn.113.184820. Epub 2014 Jan 8. PMID: 24401816; PMCID: PMC3927547.

16. Karamali M, Kashanian M, Alaeinasab S, Asemi Z. The effect of dietary soy intake on weight loss, glycaemic control, lipid profiles and biomarkers of inflammation and oxidative stress in women with polycystic ovary syndrome: a randomised clinical trial. J Hum Nutr Diet. 2018 Aug;31(4):533–543. doi: 10.1111/jhn.12545. Epub 2018 Feb 22. PMID: 29468748.

17. Haudum C, Lindheim L, Ascani A, Trummer C, Horvath A, Münzker J, Obermayer-Pietsch B. Impact of short-term isoflavone intervention in polycystic ovary syndrome (PCOS) patients on microbiota composition and metagenomics. Nutrients. 2020 Jun 1;12(6):1622. doi: 10.3390/nu12061622. PMID: 32492805; PMCID: PMC7656308.

18. Hahn KA, Wesselink AK, Wise LA, Mikkelsen EM, Cueto HT, Tucker KL, Vinceti M, Rothman KJ, Sorensen HT, Hatch EE. Iron consumption is not consistently associated with fecundability among North American and Danish pregnancy planners. J Nutr. 2019 Sep 1;149(9):1585-1595. doi: 10.1093/jn/nxz094. PMID: 31152673; PMCID: PMC6735943.

Chapter 6 References

1. Calcium. The Nutrition Source. Harvard T. H. Chan School of Public Health. www.hsph.harvard.edu/nutritionsource/what-should-you-eat/calcium-and-milk/calcium-full-story/. Accessed 9/25/23.

2. Chavarro JE, Rich-Edwards JW, Rosner B, Willett WC. A prospective study of dairy foods intake and anovulatory infertility. Hum Reprod. 2007 May;22(5):1340–1347. doi: 10.1093/humrep/dem019. Epub 2007 Feb 28. PMID: 17329264.

3. Salas-Huetos A, Bulló M, Salas-Salvadó J. Dietary patterns, foods and nutrients in male fertility parameters and fecundability: a systematic review of observational studies. Hum Reprod Update. 2017 Jul 1;23(4):371–389. doi: 10.1093/humupd/dmx006. PMID: 28333357.

4. Souter I, Chiu YH, Batsis M, Afeiche MC, Williams PL, Hauser R, Chavarro JE; EARTH Study Team. The association of protein intake (amount and type) with ovarian antral follicle counts among infertile women: results from the EARTH prospective study cohort. BJOG. 2017 Sep;124(10):1547–1555. doi: 10.1111/1471-0528.14630. Epub 2017 Apr 10. PMID: 28278351; PMCID: PMC5568942.

5. Chu J, Gallos I, Tobias A, Tan B, Eapen A, Coomarasamy A. Vitamin D and assisted reproductive treatment outcome: a systematic review and meta-analysis. Hum Reprod. 2018 Jan 1;33(1):65–80. doi: 10.1093/humrep/dex326. PMID: 29149263.

6. Ozkan S, Jindal S, Greenseid K, Shu J, Zeitlian G, Hickmon C, Pal L. Replete vitamin D stores predict reproductive success following in vitro fertilization. Fertil Steril. 2010 Sep;94(4):1314–1319. doi: 10.1016/j.fertnstert.2009.05.019. Epub 2009 Jul 8. PMID: 19589516; PMCID: PMC2888852.

7. Lerchbaum E, Rabe T. Vitamin D and female fertility. Curr Opin Obstet Gynecol. 2014 Jun;26(3):145–150. doi: 10.1097/GCO.0000000000000065. PMID: 24717915.

8. Lerchbaum E, Obermayer-Pietsch B. Vitamin D and fertility: a systematic review. Eur J Endocrinol. 2012 May;166(5):765–778. doi: 10.1530/EJE-11-0984. Epub 2012 Jan 24. PMID: 22275473.

9. Zhao J, Liu S, Wang Y, Wang P, Qu D, Liu M, Ma W, Li Y. Vitamin D improves in-vitro fertilization outcomes in infertile women with polycystic ovary syndrome and insulin resistance. Minerva Med. 2019 Jun;110(3):199–208. doi: 10.23736/S0026-4806.18.05946-3. Epub 2019 Jan 4. PMID: 30612423.

10. Blomberg Jensen M, Gerner Lawaetz J, Andersson AM, Petersen JH, Nordkap L, Bang AK, Ekbom P, Joensen UN, Prætorius L, Lundstrøm P, Boujida VH, Lanske B, Juul A, Jørgensen N. Vitamin D deficiency and low ionized calcium are linked with semen quality and sex steroid levels in infertile men. Hum Reprod. 2016 Aug;31(8):1875–1885. doi: 10.1093/humrep/dew152. Epub 2016 Jun 19. PMID: 27496946.

11. Tamblyn JA, Pilarski NSP, Markland AD, Marson EJ, Devall A, Hewison M, Morris RK, Coomarasamy A. Vitamin D and miscarriage: a systematic review and meta-analysis. Fertil Steril. 2022 Jul;118(1):111–122. doi: 10.1016/j.fertnstert.2022.04.017. Epub 2022 May 28. PMID: 35637024.

12. Várbíró S, Takács I, Tűű L, Nas K, Sziva RE, Hetthéssy JR, Török M. Effects of vitamin D on fertility, pregnancy and polycystic ovary syndrome—A review. Nutrients. 2022 Apr 15;14(8):1649. doi: 10.3390/nu14081649. PMID: 35458211; PMCID: PMC9029121.

13. Gaskins AJ, Chavarro JE. Diet and fertility: a review. Am J Obstet Gynecol. 2018 Apr;218(4):379–389. doi: 10.1016/j.ajog.2017.08.010. Epub 2017 Aug 24. PMID: 28844822; PMCID: PMC5826784.

14. Şanlier N, Gökcen BB, Sezgin AC. Health benefits of fermented foods. Crit Rev Food Sci Nutr. 2019;59(3):506–527. doi: 10.1080/10408398.2017.1383355. Epub 2017 Oct 20. PMID: 28945458.

15. Mathur H, Beresford TP, Cotter PD. Health benefits of lactic acid bacteria (LAB) fermentates. Nutrients. 2020 Jun 4;12(6):1679. doi: 10.3390/nu12061679. PMID: 32512787; PMCID: PMC7352953.

Chapter 7 References

1. Christ A, Lauterbach M, Latz E. Western diet and the immune system: An inflammatory connection. Immunity. 2019 Nov 19;51(5):794–811. doi: 10.1016/j.immuni.2019.09.020. PMID: 31747581.

2. Cancer: Carcinogenicity of the consumption of red meat and processed meats. Questions and Answers. World Health Organization, October 26, 2015. www.who.int/news-room/questions-and-answers /item/cancer-carcinogenicity-of-the-consumption-of-red-meat-and-processed-meat.

3. Zhong VW, Van Horn L, Greenland P, Carnethon MR, Ning H, Wilkins JT, Lloyd-Jones DM, Allen NB. Associations of processed meat, unprocessed red meat, poultry, or fish intake with incident cardiovascular disease and all-cause mortality. JAMA Intern Med. 2020 Apr 1;180(4):503–512. doi: 10.1001/jamainternmed.2019.6969. PMID: 32011623; PMCID: PMC7042891.

4. Chavarro JE, Rich-Edwards JW, Rosner BA, Willett WC. Diet and lifestyle in the prevention of ovulatory disorder infertility. Obstet Gynecol. 2007 Nov;110(5):1050–1058. doi: 10.1097/01 .AOG.0000287293.25465.e1. PMID: 17978119.

5. Karayiannis D, Kontogianni MD, Mendorou C, Mastrominas M, Yiannakouris N. Adherence to the Mediterranean diet and IVF success rate among non-obese women attempting fertility. Hum Reprod. 2018 Mar 1;33(3):494–502. doi: 10.1093/humrep/dey003. PMID: 29390148.

6. Gaskins AJ, Nassan FL, Chiu YH, Arvizu M, Williams PL, Keller MG, Souter I, Hauser R, Chavarro JE; EARTH Study Team. Dietary patterns and outcomes of assisted reproduction. Am J Obstet Gynecol. 2019 Jun;220(6):567.e1–567.e18. doi: 10.1016/j.ajog.2019.02.004. Epub 2019 Feb 8. PMID: 30742825; PMCID: PMC6545142.

7. Braga DP, Halpern G, Setti AS, Figueira RC, Iaconelli A Jr, Borges E Jr. The impact of food intake and social habits on embryo quality and the likelihood of blastocyst formation. Reprod Biomed Online (2015) 31:30–38. doi: 10.1016/j.rbmo.2015.03.007.

8. Attaman JA, Toth TL, Furtado J, Campos H, Hauser R, Chavarro JE. Dietary fat and semen quality among men attending a fertility clinic. Hum Reprod. (2012) 27:1466–1474. doi: 10.1093 /humrep/des065.

9. Salas-Huetos A, Bulló M, Salas-Salvadó J. Dietary patterns, foods and nutrients in male fertility parameters and fecundability: a systematic review of observational studies. Hum Reprod Update. 2017 Jul 1;23(4):371–389. doi: 10.1093/humupd/dmx006. PMID: 28333357.

10. Chavarro JE, Rich-Edwards JW, Rosner BA, Willett WC. Protein intake and ovulatory infertility. Am J Obstet Gynecol. 2008 Feb;198(2):210.e1–7. doi: 10.1016/j.ajog.2007.06.057. PMID: 18226626; PMCID: PMC3066040.

11. Xia W, Chiu YH, Williams PL, Gaskins AJ, Toth TL, Tanrikut C, Hauser R, Chavarro JE. Men's meat intake and treatment outcomes among couples undergoing assisted reproduction. Fertil Steril. 2015 Oct;104(4):972–979. doi: 10.1016/j.fertnstert.2015.06.037. Epub 2015 Jul 20. PMID: 26206344; PMCID: PMC4592805.

12. Uribarri J, Woodruff S, Goodman S, Cai W, Chen X, Pyzik R, Yong A, Striker GE, Vlassara H. Advanced glycation end products in foods and a practical guide to their reduction in the diet. J Am Diet Assoc. 2010 Jun;110(6):911–916.e12. doi: 10.1016/j.jada.2010.03.018. PMID: 20497781; PMCID: PMC3704564.

13. Ruiz HH, Ramasamy R, Schmidt AM. Advanced glycation end products: Building on the concept of the "common soil" in metabolic disease. Endocrinology. 2020 Jan 1;161(1):bqz006. doi: 10.1210 /endocr/bqz006. PMID: 31638645; PMCID: PMC7188081.

14. Muthyalaiah YS, Jonnalagadda B, John CM, Arockiasamy S. Impact of Advanced Glycation End products (AGEs) and its receptor (RAGE) on cancer metabolic signaling pathways and its

progression. Glycoconj J. 2021 Dec;38(6):717–734. doi: 10.1007/s10719-021-10031-x. Epub 2022 Jan 22. PMID: 35064413.

15. Tantalaki E, Piperi C, Livadas S, Kollias A, Adamopoulos C, Koulouri A, Christakou C, Diamanti-Kandarakis E. Impact of dietary modification of advanced glycation end products (AGEs) on the hormonal and metabolic profile of women with polycystic ovary syndrome (PCOS). Hormones (Athens). 2014 Jan-Mar;13(1):65–73. doi: 10.1007/BF03401321. PMID: 24722128.

16. Merhi Z, Mcgee EA, Buyuk E. Role of advanced glycation end-products in obesity-related ovarian dysfunction. Minerva Endocrinol. 2014 Sep;39(3):167–174. PMID: 25068304.

17. Ólafsson, Björn. Is beef consumption headed in the right direction? Sentient Media, April 26, 2023. https://sentientmedia.org/beef-consumption-in-the-us/.

18. Meyer N, Reguant-Closa A. "Eat as if you could save the planet and win!" Sustainability integration into nutrition for exercise and sport. Nutrients. 2017 Apr 21;9(4):412. doi: 10.3390/nu9040412. PMID: 28430140; PMCID: PMC5409751.

19. Culinary Institute of America. The CIA Challenges Chefs to Rethink the "Protein Portfolio" on their Menus. www.ciachef.edu/protein-portfolio-release/. Accessed 10/2/2023.

20. Päivärinta E, Itkonen ST, Pellinen T, Lehtovirta M, Erkkola M, Pajari AM. Replacing animal-based proteins with plant-based proteins changes the composition of a whole Nordic diet: A randomised clinical trial in healthy Finnish adults. Nutrients. 2020 Mar 28;12(4):943. doi: 10.3390/nu12040943. PMID: 32231103; PMCID: PMC7231027.

21. Meyer N, Reguant-Closa A. "Eat as if you could save the planet and win!" Sustainability integration into nutrition for exercise and sport. Nutrients. 2017 Apr 21;9(4):412. doi: 10.3390/nu9040412. PMID: 28430140; PMCID: PMC5409751.

22. Fouillet H, Dussiot A, Perraud E, Wang J, Huneau JF, Kesse-Guyot E, Mariotti F. Plant to animal protein ratio in the diet: nutrient adequacy, long-term health and environmental pressure. Front Nutr. 2023 Jun 15;10:1178121. doi: 10.3389/fnut.2023.1178121. Erratum in: Front Nutr. 2023 Sep 01;10:1281700. PMID: 37396122; PMCID: PMC10311446.

Chapter 8 References

1. Pulver, Jeffrey R., Alan Lowther, and Melissa A. Yencho. 2020. Updating the NOAA Fisheries Per Capita Consumption Model. NOAA Tech. Memo. NMFS-F/SPO-210, 24 p. 13.

2. Krittanawong C, Isath A, Hahn J, Wang Z, Narasimhan B, Kaplin SL, Jneid H, Virani SS, Tang WHW. Fish consumption and cardiovascular health: A systematic review. Am J Med. 2021 Jun;134(6):713–720. doi: 10.1016/j.amjmed.2020.12.017. Epub 2021 Jan 11. PMID: 33444594.

3. Mozaffarian D, Rimm EB. Fish intake, contaminants, and human health: evaluating the risks and the benefits. JAMA. 2006 Oct 18;296(15):1885-99. doi: 10.1001/jama.296.15.1885. Erratum in: JAMA. 2007 Feb 14;297(6):590. PMID: 17047219.

4. Gaskins AJ, Sundaram R, Buck Louis GM, Chavarro JE. Seafood intake, sexual activity, and time to pregnancy. J Clin Endocrinol Metab. 2018 Jul 1;103(7):2680–2688. doi: 10.1210/jc.2018-00385. PMID: 29800287; PMCID: PMC6276709.

5. Toledo E, Lopez-del Burgo C, Ruiz-Zambrana A, Donazar M, Navarro-Blasco I, Martínez-González MA, de Irala J. Dietary patterns and difficulty conceiving: a nested case-control study. Fertil Steril. 2011 Nov;96(5):1149–53. doi: 10.1016/j.fertnstert.2011.08.034. Epub 2011 Sep 22. PMID: 21943725.

6. Afeiche MC, Gaskins AJ, Williams PL, Toth TL, Wright DL, Tanrikut C, Hauser R, Chavarro JE. Processed meat intake is unfavorably and fish intake favorably associated with semen quality indicators among men attending a fertility clinic. J Nutr. 2014 Jul;144(7):1091–1098. doi: 10.3945/jn.113.190173. Epub 2014 May 21. PMID: 24850626; PMCID: PMC4056648.

7. Braga DP, Halpern G, Setti AS, Figueira RC, Iaconelli A Jr, Borges E Jr. The impact of food intake and social habits on embryo quality and the likelihood of blastocyst formation. Reprod Biomed Online. 2015 Jul;31(1):30–38. doi: 10.1016/j.rbmo.2015.03.007. Epub 2015 Mar 27. PMID: 25982093.

8. Nassan FL, Chiu YH, Vanegas JC, Gaskins AJ, Williams PL, Ford JB, Attaman J, Hauser R, Chavarro JE; EARTH Study Team. Intake of protein-rich foods in relation to outcomes of infertility treatment with assisted reproductive technologies. Am J Clin Nutr. 2018 Nov 1;108(5):1104–1112. doi: 10.1093/ajcn/nqy185. PMID: 30475972; PMCID: PMC6692709.

9. Chiu YH, Karmon AE, Gaskins AJ, Arvizu M, Williams PL, Souter I, Rueda BR, Hauser R, Chavarro JE; EARTH Study Team. Serum omega-3 fatty acids and treatment outcomes among women undergoing assisted reproduction. Hum Reprod. 2018 Jan 1;33(1):156–165. doi: 10.1093/humrep/dex335. PMID: 29136189; PMCID: PMC5850735.

10. Hammiche F, Vujkovic M, Wijburg W, de Vries JH, Macklon NS, Laven JS, Steegers-Theunissen RP. Increased preconception omega-3 polyunsaturated fatty acid intake improves embryo morphology. Fertil Steril. 2011 Apr;95(5):1820–1823. doi: 10.1016/j.fertnstert.2010.11.021. Epub 2010 Dec 3. PMID: 21130435.

11. Wise LA, Willis SK, Mikkelsen EM, Wesselink AK, Sørensen HT, Rothman KJ, Tucker KL, Trolle E, Vinceti M, Hatch EE. The association between seafood intake and fecundability: Analysis from two prospective studies. Nutrients. 2020 Jul 29;12(8):2276. doi: 10.3390/nu12082276. PMID: 32751290; PMCID: PMC7469023.

12. Kimáková T, Kuzmová L, Nevolná Z, Bencko V. Fish and fish products as risk factors of mercury exposure. Ann Agric Environ Med. 2018 Sep 25;25(3):488–493. doi: 10.26444/aaem/84934. Epub 2018 Mar 23. PMID: 30260185.

13. Gil A, Gil F. Fish, a Mediterranean source of n-3 PUFA: benefits do not justify limiting consumption. Br J Nutr. 2015 Apr;113 Suppl 2:S58–67. doi: 10.1017/S0007114514003742. PMID: 26148923.

14. American College of Obstetricians and Gynecologists. ACOG Practice advisory: update on seafood consumption during pregnancy. 2017. Available at: www.acog.org/Clinical-Guidance-and-Publications/Practice-Advisories/ACOG-Practice-Advisory-Seafood-Consumption-During-Pregnancy.

15. Advice about eating fish for those who might become or are pregnant or breastfeeding and children ages 1–11 years. U.S. Food & Drug Administration, revised September 28, 2022. www.FDA.gov/fishadvice. Accessed 9/25/2023.

16. Healthy fish guide. Washington State Department of Health. doh.wa.gov/community-and -environment/food/fish/healthy-fish-guide. Accessed 9/25/2023.

17. Mozaffarian D, Rimm EB. Fish intake, contaminants, and human health: Evaluating the risks and the benefits. JAMA. 2006 Oct 18;296(15):1885–1899. doi: 10.1001/jama.296.15.1885. Erratum in: JAMA. 2007 Feb 14;297(6):590. PMID: 17047219.

18. Consumer guides. Monterey Bay Aquarium Seafood Watch. www.seafoodwatch.org/recommendations /download-consumer-guides.

19. Hibbeln JR, Davis JM, Steer C, Emmett P, Rogers I, Williams C, Golding J. Maternal seafood consumption in pregnancy and neurodevelopmental outcomes in childhood (ALSPAC study): An observational cohort study. Lancet. 2007 Feb 17;369(9561):578–585. doi: 10.1016/S0140-6736(07)60277-3. PMID: 17307104.

Chapter 9 References

1. Willett WC, Stampfer MJ, Manson JE, Colditz GA, Speizer FE, Rosner BA, Sampson LA, Hennekens CH. Intake of trans fatty acids and risk of coronary heart disease among women. Lancet. 1993 Mar 6;341(8845):581–585. doi: 10.1016/0140-6736(93)90350-p. PMID: 8094827.

2. Amico A, Wootan MG, Jacobson MF, Leung C, Willett AW. The demise of artificial trans fat: A history of a public health achievement. Milbank Q. 2021 Sep;99(3):746–770. doi: 10.1111/1468 -0009.12515. Epub 2021 Aug 3. PMID: 34342900; PMCID: PMC8452362.

3. Satija A, Bhupathiraju SN, Spiegelman D, Chiuve SE, Manson JE, Willett W, Rexrode KM, Rimm EB, Hu FB. Healthful and unhealthful plant-based diets and the risk of coronary heart disease in U.S. adults. J Am Coll Cardiol. 2017 Jul 25;70(4):411–422. doi: 10.1016/j.jacc.2017.05.047. PMID: 28728684; PMCID: PMC5555375.

4. Guasch-Ferré M, Zong G, Willett WC, Zock PL, Wanders AJ, Hu FB, Sun Q. Associations of monounsaturated fatty acids from plant and animal sources with total and cause-specific mortality in two US prospective cohort studies. Circ Res. 2019 Apr 12;124(8):1266–1275. doi: 10.1161 /CIRCRESAHA.118.313996. PMID: 30689516; PMCID: PMC6459723.

5. Hu FB, Willett WC. Diet and coronary heart disease: Findings from the Nurses' Health Study and Health Professionals' Follow-up Study. J Nutr Health Aging. 2001;5(3):132–138. PMID: 11458281.

6. Ericson U, Hellstrand S, Brunkwall L, Schulz CA, Sonestedt E, Wallström P, Gullberg B, Wirfält E, Orho-Melander M. Food sources of fat may clarify the inconsistent role of dietary fat intake for incidence of type 2 diabetes. Am J Clin Nutr. 2015 May;101(5):1065–1080. doi: 10.3945 /ajcn.114.103010. Epub 2015 Apr 1. PMID: 25832335.

7. Guasch-Ferré M, Becerra-Tomás N, Ruiz-Canela M, Corella D, Schröder H, Estruch R, Ros E, Arós F, Gómez-Gracia E, Fiol M, Serra-Majem L, Lapetra J, Basora J, Martín-Calvo N, Portoles O, Fitó M, Hu FB, Forga L, Salas-Salvadó J. Total and subtypes of dietary fat intake and risk of type 2 diabetes mellitus in the Prevención con Dieta Mediterránea (PREDIMED) study. Am J Clin Nutr. 2017 Mar;105(3):723–735. doi: 10.3945/ajcn.116.142034. Epub 2017 Feb 15. PMID: 28202478.

8. Chiu YH, Karmon AE, Gaskins AJ, Arvizu M, Williams PL, Souter I, Rueda BR, Hauser R, Chavarro JE; EARTH Study Team. Serum omega-3 fatty acids and treatment outcomes among women undergoing assisted reproduction. Hum Reprod. 2018 Jan 1;33(1):156–165. doi: 10.1093/humrep /dex335. PMID: 29136189; PMCID: PMC5850735.

9. Hammiche F, Vujkovic M, Wijburg W, de Vries JH, Macklon NS, Laven JS, Steegers-Theunissen RP. Increased preconception omega-3 polyunsaturated fatty acid intake improves embryo morphology. Fertil Steril. 2011 Apr;95(5):1820–1823. doi: 10.1016/j.fertnstert.2010.11.021. Epub 2010 Dec 3. PMID: 21130435.

10. Hohos NM, Skaznik-Wikiel ME. High-fat diet and female fertility. Endocrinology. 2017 Aug 1;158(8):2407–2419. doi: 10.1210/en.2017-00371. PMID: 28586412; PMCID: PMC6283234.

11. Nehra D, Le HD, Fallon EM, Carlson SJ, Woods D, White YA, Pan AH, Guo L, Rodig SJ, Tilly JL, Rueda BR, Puder M. Prolonging the female reproductive lifespan and improving egg quality with dietary omega-3 fatty acids. Aging Cell. 2012 Dec;11(6):1046-54. doi: 10.1111/acel.12006. Epub 2012 Oct 19. PMID: 22978268; PMCID: PMC5624332.

12. Skoracka K, Eder P, Łykowska-Szuber L, Dobrowolska A, Krela-Kaźmierczak I. Diet and nutritional factors in male (in)fertility-underestimated factors. J Clin Med. 2020 May 9;9(5):1400. doi: 10.3390/jcm9051400. PMID: 32397485; PMCID: PMC7291266.

13. Grieger JA, Grzeskowiak LE, Wilson RL, Bianco-Miotto T, Leemaqz SY, Jankovic-Karasoulos T, Perkins AV, Norman RJ, Dekker GA, Roberts CT. Maternal selenium, copper and zinc concentrations in early pregnancy, and the association with fertility. Nutrients. 2019 Jul 16;11(7):1609. doi: 10.3390/nu11071609. PMID: 31315178; PMCID: PMC6683068.

14. Brigelius-Flohé R, Maiorino M. Glutathione peroxidases. Biochim Biophys Acta. 2013 May;1830(5):3289–3303. doi: 10.1016/j.bbagen.2012.11.020. Epub 2012 Nov 29. PMID: 23201771.

15. Lima LG, Santos AAMD, Gueiber TD, Gomes RZ, Martins CM, Chaikoski AC. Relation between selenium and female fertility: A systematic review. Rev Bras Ginecol Obstet. 2022 Jun 3. English. doi: 10.1055/s-0042-1744288. Epub ahead of print. PMID: 35668679.

16. Köhrle J. Selenium and the thyroid. Curr Opin Endocrinol Diabetes Obes. 2015 Oct;22(5):392–401. doi: 10.1097/MED.0000000000000190. PMID: 26313901.

17. Jiang TA. Health benefits of culinary herbs and spices. J AOAC Int. 2019 Mar 1;102(2):395–411. doi: 10.5740/jaoacint.18-0418. Epub 2019 Jan 16. PMID: 30651162.

18. Opara EI, Chohan M. Culinary herbs and spices: their bioactive properties, the contribution of polyphenols and the challenges in deducing their true health benefits. Int J Mol Sci. 2014 Oct 22;15(10):19183–19202. doi: 10.3390/ijms151019183. PMID: 25340982; PMCID: PMC4227268.

19. Bengmark S, Mesa MD, Gil A. Plant-derived health: the effects of turmeric and curcuminoids. Nutr Hosp. 2009 May–Jun;24(3):273–281. PMID: 19721899.

20. Krishnaswamy K. Traditional Indian spices and their health significance. Asia Pac J Clin Nutr. 2008;17 Suppl 1:265–268. PMID: 18296352.

21. Percival SS, Vanden Heuvel JP, Nieves CJ, Montero C, Migliaccio AJ, Meadors J. Bioavailability of herbs and spices in humans as determined by ex vivo inflammatory suppression and DNA strand breaks. J Am Coll Nutr. 2012 Aug;31(4):288–294. doi: 10.1080/07315724.2012.10720438. PMID: 23378457.

22. Jessica Elizabeth T, Gassara F, Kouassi AP, Brar SK, Belkacemi K. Spice use in food: Properties and benefits. Crit Rev Food Sci Nutr. 2017 Apr 13;57(6):1078–1088. doi: 10.1080/10408398.2013.858235. PMID: 26560460.

23. Bower A, Marquez S, de Mejia EG. The health benefits of selected culinary herbs and spices found in the traditional Mediterranean diet. Crit Rev Food Sci Nutr. 2016 Dec 9;56(16):2728–2746. doi: 10.1080/10408398.2013.805713. PMID: 25749238.

24. Tapsell LC, Hemphill I, Cobiac L, Patch CS, Sullivan DR, Fenech M, Roodenrys S, Keogh JB, Clifton PM, Williams PG, Fazio VA, Inge KE. Health benefits of herbs and spices: the past, the present, the future. Med J Aust. 2006 Aug 21;185(S4):S1–S24. doi: 10.5694/j.1326-5377.2006.tb00548.x. PMID: 17022438.

Chapter 10 References

1. Zong G, Eisenberg DM, Hu FB, Sun Q. Consumption of meals prepared at home and risk of type 2 diabetes: An analysis of two prospective cohort studies. PLoS Med. 2016 Jul 5;13(7):e1002052. doi: 10.1371/journal.pmed.1002052. PMID: 27379673; PMCID: PMC4933392.

2. Hemilä H, Chalker E. Vitamin C for preventing and treating the common cold. Cochrane Database Syst Rev. 2013 Jan 31;2013(1):CD000980. doi: 10.1002/14651858.CD000980.pub4. PMID: 23440782; PMCID: PMC8078152.

3. Should we prescribe calcium or vitamin D supplements to treat or prevent osteoporosis? Climacteric. 2015;18 Suppl 2:22–31. doi: 10.3109/13697137.2015.1098266. Epub 2015 Oct 16. PMID: 26473773.

4. Gaskins AJ, Rich-Edwards JW, Hauser R, Williams PL, Gillman MW, Ginsburg ES, Missmer SA, Chavarro JE. Maternal prepregnancy folate intake and risk of spontaneous abortion and stillbirth. Obstet Gynecol. 2014 Jul;124(1):23–31. doi: 10.1097/AOG.0000000000000343. PMID: 24901281; PMCID: PMC4086728.

5. Practice Bulletin No. 187 Summary: Neural Tube Defects. Obstet Gynecol. 2017 Dec;130(6):1394–1396. doi: 10.1097/AOG.0000000000002410. PMID: 29189691.

6. Kennedy D, Koren G. Identifying women who might benefit from higher doses of folic acid in pregnancy. Can Fam Physician. 2012 Apr;58(4):394–397. PMID: 22499814; PMCID: PMC3325450.

7. Dwyer ER, Filion KB, MacFarlane AJ, Platt RW, Mehrabadi A. Who should consume high-dose folic acid supplements before and during early pregnancy for the prevention of neural tube defects? BMJ. 2022 Jun 7;377:e067728. doi: 10.1136/bmj-2021-067728. PMID: 35672044.

8. MTHFR gene, folic acid, and preventing neural tube defects. Folic Acid. Centers for Disease Control and Prevention. https://www.cdc.gov/ncbddd/folicacid/mthfr-gene-and-folic-acid.html. Accessed on 9/26/2023.

9. Lee SY, Stagnaro-Green A, MacKay D, Wong AW, Pearce EN. Iodine contents in prenatal vitamins in the United States. Thyroid. 2017 Aug;27(8):1101–1102. doi: 10.1089/thy.2017.0097. Epub 2017 Jul 11. PMID: 28599614; PMCID: PMC5912719.

10. Gaskins AJ, Nassan FL, Chiu YH, Arvizu M, Williams PL, Keller MG, Souter I, Hauser R, Chavarro JE; EARTH Study Team. Dietary patterns and outcomes of assisted reproduction. Am J

Obstet Gynecol. 2019 Jun;220(6):567.e1–567.e18. doi: 10.1016/j.ajog.2019.02.004. Epub 2019 Feb 8. PMID: 30742825; PMCID: PMC6545142.

11. Chu J, Gallos I, Tobias A, Tan B, Eapen A, Coomarasamy A. Vitamin D and assisted reproductive treatment outcome: a systematic review and meta-analysis. Hum Reprod. 2018 Jan 1;33(1):65–80. doi: 10.1093/humrep/dex326. PMID: 29149263.

12. Zhao J, Huang X, Xu B, Yan Y, Zhang Q, Li Y. Whether vitamin D was associated with clinical outcome after IVF/ICSI: a systematic review and meta-analysis. Reprod Biol Endocrinol. 2018 Feb 9;16(1):13. doi: 10.1186/s12958-018-0324-3. PMID: 29426322; PMCID: PMC5807754.

13. Tamblyn JA, Pilarski NSP, Markland AD, Marson EJ, Devall A, Hewison M, Morris RK, Coomarasamy A. Vitamin D and miscarriage: a systematic review and meta-analysis. Fertil Steril. 2022 Jul;118(1):111–122. doi: 10.1016/j.fertnstert.2022.04.017. Epub 2022 May 28. PMID: 35637024.

14. Palacios C, Kostiuk LK, Peña-Rosas JP. Vitamin D supplementation for women during pregnancy. Cochrane Database Syst Rev. 2019 Jul 26;7(7):CD008873. doi: 10.1002/14651858.CD008873.pub4. PMID: 31348529; PMCID: PMC6659840.

15. Showell MG, Mackenzie-Proctor R, Jordan V, Hart RJ. Antioxidants for female subfertility. Cochrane Database Syst Rev. 2020 Aug 27;8(8):CD007807. doi: 10.1002/14651858.CD007807.pub4. PMID: 32851663; PMCID: PMC8094745.

16. de Ligny W, Smits RM, Mackenzie-Proctor R, Jordan V, Fleischer K, de Bruin JP, Showell MG. Antioxidants for male subfertility. Cochrane Database Syst Rev. 2022 May 4;5(5):CD007411. doi: 10.1002/14651858.CD007411.pub5. PMID: 35506389; PMCID: PMC9066298.

17. Zhang M, ShiYang X, Zhang Y, Miao Y, Chen Y, Cui Z, Xiong B. Coenzyme Q10 ameliorates the quality of postovulatory aged oocytes by suppressing DNA damage and apoptosis. Free Radic Biol Med. 2019 Nov 1;143:84–94. doi: 10.1016/j.freeradbiomed.2019.08.002. Epub 2019 Aug 6. PMID: 31398498.

18. Ben-Meir A, Burstein E, Borrego-Alvarez A, Chong J, Wong E, Yavorska T, Naranian T, Chi M, Wang Y, Bentov Y, Alexis J, Meriano J, Sung HK, Gasser DL, Moley KH, Hekimi S, Casper RF, Jurisicova A. Coenzyme Q10 restores oocyte mitochondrial function and fertility during reproductive aging. Aging Cell. 2015 Oct;14(5):887–895. doi: 10.1111/acel.12368. Epub 2015 Jun 26. PMID: 26111777; PMCID: PMC4568976.

19. Rodríguez-Varela C, Labarta E. Does Coenzyme Q10 supplementation improve human oocyte quality? Int J Mol Sci. 2021 Sep 2;22(17):9541. doi: 10.3390/ijms22179541. PMID: 34502447; PMCID: PMC8431086.

20. Florou P, Anagnostis P, Theocharis P, Chourdakis M, Goulis DG. Does coenzyme Q10 supplementation improve fertility outcomes in women undergoing assisted reproductive technology procedures? A systematic review and meta-analysis of randomized-controlled trials. J Assist Reprod Genet. 2020 Oct;37(10):2377–2387. doi: 10.1007/s10815-020-01906-3. Epub 2020 Aug 7. PMID: 32767206; PMCID: PMC7550497.

21. Mancini A, Balercia G. Coenzyme Q(10) in male infertility: physiopathology and therapy. Biofactors. 2011 Sep–Oct;37(5):374–380. doi: 10.1002/biof.164. Epub 2011 Oct 11. PMID: 21989906. Studies have failed to show that supplementation leads to increased pregnancy rates.

22. Sharma AP, Sharma G, Kumar R. Systematic review and meta-analysis on effect of carnitine, co-enzyme Q10 and selenium on pregnancy and semen parameters in couples with idiopathic male infertility. Urology. 2022 Mar;161:4–11. doi: 10.1016/j.urology.2021.10.041. Epub 2021 Dec 4. PMID: 34871624.

23. Greff D, Juhász AE, Váncsa S, Váradi A, Sipos Z, Szinte J, Park S, Hegyi P, Nyirády P, Ács N, Várbíró S, Horváth EM. Inositol is an effective and safe treatment in polycystic ovary syndrome: a systematic review and meta-analysis of randomized controlled trials. Reprod Biol Endocrinol. 2023 Jan 26;21(1):10. doi: 10.1186/s12958-023-01055-z. PMID: 36703143; PMCID: PMC9878965.

24. Menichini D, Facchinetti F. Effects of vitamin D supplementation in women with polycystic ovary syndrome: A review. Gynecol Endocrinol. 2020 Jan;36(1):1–5. doi: 10.1080/09513590.2019.1625881. Epub 2019 Jun 12. PMID: 31187648.

25. Chavarro JE, Rich-Edwards JW, Rosner BA, Willett WC. Iron intake and risk of ovulatory infertility. Obstet Gynecol. 2006 Nov;108(5):1145–1152. doi: 10.1097/01.AOG.0000238333.37423.ab. PMID: 17077236.

26. Samimi M, Zarezade Mehrizi M, Foroozanfard F, Akbari H, Jamilian M, Ahmadi S, Asemi Z. The effects of coenzyme Q10 supplementation on glucose metabolism and lipid profiles in women with polycystic ovary syndrome: A randomized, double-blind, placebo-controlled trial. Clin Endocrinol (Oxf). 2017 Apr;86(4):560–566. doi: 10.1111/cen.13288. Epub 2017 Jan 10. PMID: 27911471.

Chapter 11 References

1. Mena GP, Mielke GI, Brown WJ. The effect of physical activity on reproductive health outcomes in young women: a systematic review and meta-analysis. Hum Reprod Update. 2019 Sep 11;25(5):541–563. doi: 10.1093/humupd/dmz013. PMID: 31304974.

2. Wise LA, Rothman KJ, Mikkelsen EM, Sørensen HT, Riis AH, Hatch EE. A prospective cohort study of physical activity and time to pregnancy. Fertil Steril. 2012 May;97(5):1136–1142.e1-4. doi: 10.1016/j.fertnstert.2012.02.025. Epub 2012 Mar 15. PMID: 22425198; PMCID: PMC3340509.

3. Woodward A, Klonizakis M, Broom D. Exercise and polycystic ovary syndrome. Adv Exp Med Biol. 2020;1228:123–136. doi: 10.1007/978-981-15-1792-1_8. PMID: 32342454.

4. Ibid.

5. Wright PJ, Corbett CF, Pinto BM, Dawson RM, Wirth M. Resistance training as therapeutic management in women with PCOS: What is the evidence? Int J Exerc Sci. 2021 Aug 1;14(3):840–854. PMID: 34567361; PMCID: PMC8439708.

6. Hakimi O, Cameron LC. Effect of exercise on ovulation: A systematic review. Sports Med. 2017 Aug;47(8):1555–1567. doi: 10.1007/s40279-016-0669-8. PMID: 28035585., Huhmann K. Menses requires energy: A review of how disordered eating, excessive exercise, and high stress lead to menstrual irregularities. Clin Ther. 2020 Mar;42(3):401–407. doi: 10.1016/j.clinthera.2020.01.016. Epub 2020 Mar 2. PMID: 32139174.

7. Rinaldi, Nicola. *No Period, Now What?* Waltham, MA: Antica Press, 2019.

8. Memme JM, Erlich AT, Phukan G, Hood DA. Exercise and mitochondrial health. J Physiol. 2021 Feb;599(3):803–817. doi: 10.1113/JP278853. Epub 2019 Dec 9. PMID: 31674658.

9. Mitchell R. Is physical activity in natural environments better for mental health than physical activity in other environments? Soc Sci Med. 2013 Aug;91:130–134. doi: 10.1016/j.socscimed .2012.04.012. Epub 2012 May 8. PMID: 22705180.

10. Lahart I, Darcy P, Gidlow C, Calogiuri G. The effects of green exercise on physical and mental well-being: A systematic review. Int J Environ Res Public Health. 2019 Apr 15;16(8):1352. doi: 10.3390 /ijerph16081352. PMID: 30991724; PMCID: PMC6518264.

11. Park BJ, Tsunetsugu Y, Kasetani T, Kagawa T, Miyazaki Y. The physiological effects of Shin-rin-yoku (taking in the forest atmosphere or forest bathing): evidence from field experiments in 24 forests across Japan. These benefits were seen in the forest, but not in an urban environment during a crossover study. Environ Health Prev Med. 2010 Jan;15(1):18–26. doi: 10.1007/s12199 -009-0086-9. PMID: 19568835; PMCID: PMC2793346.

12. Antonelli M, Barbieri G, Donelli D. Effects of forest bathing (shinrin-yoku) on levels of cortisol as a stress biomarker: A systematic review and meta-analysis. Int J Biometeorol. 2019 Aug;63(8):1117–1134. doi: 10.1007/s00484-019-01717-x. Epub 2019 Apr 18. PMID: 31001682.

13. White MP, Alcock I, Grellier J, Wheeler BW, Hartig T, Warber SL, Bone A, Depledge MH, Fleming LE. Spending at least 120 minutes a week in nature is associated with good health and wellbeing. Sci Rep. 2019 Jun 13;9(1):7730. doi: 10.1038/s41598-019-44097-3. PMID: 31197192; PMCID: PMC6565732.

14. DiPietro L, Gribok A, Stevens MS, Hamm LF, Rumpler W. Three 15-min sessions of moderate post meal walking significantly improves 24-h glycemic control in people at risk for impaired glucose tolerance. Diabetes Care. 2013 Oct;36(10):3262–3268. doi: 10.2337/dc13-0084. Epub 2013 Jun 11. PMID: 23761134; PMCID: PMC3781561.

15. Katy Milkman. *How to Change: The Science of Getting from Where You Are to Where You Want to Be.* Portfolio; 2021.

16. Rooney KL, Domar AD. The relationship between stress and infertility. Dialogues Clin Neurosci. 2018 Mar;20(1):41–47. doi: 10.31887/DCNS.2018.20.1/klrooney. PMID: 29946210; PMCID: PMC6016043.

17. Lynch CD, Sundaram R, Maisog JM, Sweeney AM, Buck Louis GM. Preconception stress increases the risk of infertility: Results from a couple-based prospective cohort study--the LIFE study. Hum Reprod. 2014 May;29(5):1067–1075. doi: 10.1093/humrep/deu032. Epub 2014 Mar 23. PMID: 24664130; PMCID: PMC3984126.

18. Ebbesen SM, Zachariae R, Mehlsen MY, Thomsen D, Højgaard A, Ottosen L, Petersen T, Ingerslev HJ. Stressful life events are associated with a poor in-vitro fertilization (IVF) outcome: A prospective study. Hum Reprod. 2009 Sep;24(9):2173–2182. doi: 10.1093/humrep/dep185. Epub 2009 May 22. PMID: 19465459.

19. Massey AJ, Campbell BK, Raine-Fenning N, Pincott-Allen C, Perry J, Vedhara K. Relationship between hair and salivary cortisol and pregnancy in women undergoing IVF. Psychoneuroendocrinology. 2016 Dec;74:397–405. doi: 10.1016/j.psyneuen.2016.08.027. Epub 2016 Aug 31. PMID: 27756033.

20. Boivin J, Griffiths E, Venetis CA. Emotional distress in infertile women and failure of assisted reproductive technologies: Meta-analysis of prospective psychosocial studies. BMJ. 2011 Feb 23;342:d223. doi: 10.1136/bmj.d223. PMID: 21345903; PMCID: PMC3043530.

21. Luk BHK, Loke AY. Sexual satisfaction, intimacy and relationship of couples undergoing infertility treatment. J Reprod Infant Psychol. 2019 Apr;37(2):108–122. doi: 10.1080/02646838.2018.1529407. Epub 2018 Oct 15. PMID: 30317866.

22. Campagne DM. Should fertilization treatment start with reducing stress? Hum Reprod. 2006 Jul;21(7):1651–1658. doi: 10.1093/humrep/del078. Epub 2006 Mar 16. PMID: 16543257.

23. Katyal N, Poulsen CM, Knudsen UB, Frederiksen Y. The association between psychosocial interventions and fertility treatment outcome: A systematic review and meta-analysis. Eur J Obstet Gynecol Reprod Biol. 2021 Apr;259:125–132. doi: 10.1016/j.ejogrb.2021.02.012. Epub 2021 Feb 19. PMID: 33677371.

24. Gaitzsch H, Benard J, Hugon-Rodin J, Benzakour L, Streuli I. The effect of mind-body interventions on psychological and pregnancy outcomes in infertile women: a systematic review. Arch Womens Ment Health. 2020 Aug;23(4):479–491. doi: 10.1007/s00737-019-01009-8. Epub 2020 Jan 2. PMID: 31897607.

25. Domar AD, Rooney KL, Wiegand B, Orav EJ, Alper MM, Berger BM, Nikolovski J. Impact of a group mind/body intervention on pregnancy rates in IVF patients. Fertil Steril. 2011 Jun;95(7):2269–2273. doi: 10.1016/j.fertnstert.2011.03.046. Epub 2011 Apr 15. PMID: 21496800.

26. Frederiksen Y, O'Toole MS, Mehlsen MY, Hauge B, Elbaek HO, Zachariae R, Ingerslev HJ. The effect of expressive writing intervention for infertile couples: A randomized controlled trial. Hum Reprod. 2017 Feb;32(2):391–402. doi: 10.1093/humrep/dew320. Epub 2016 Dec 21. PMID: 28007790.

27. Li J, Long L, Liu Y, He W, Li M. Effects of a mindfulness-based intervention on fertility quality of life and pregnancy rates among women subjected to first in vitro fertilization treatment. Behav Res Ther. 2016 Feb;77:96–104. doi: 10.1016/j.brat.2015.12.010. Epub 2015 Dec 19. PMID: 26742022.

28. Feder A, Nestler EJ, Charney DS. Psychobiology and molecular genetics of resilience. Nat Rev Neurosci. 2009 Jun;10(6):446–457. doi: 10.1038/nrn2649. PMID: 19455174; PMCID: PMC2833107.

29. Kalsbeek A, la Fleur S, Fliers E. Circadian control of glucose metabolism. Mol Metab. 2014 Mar 19;3(4):372–383. doi: 10.1016/j.molmet.2014.03.002. PMID: 24944897; PMCID: PMC4060304.

30. Fernandez RC, Moore VM, Van Ryswyk EM, Varcoe TJ, Rodgers RJ, March WA, Moran LJ, Avery JC, McEvoy RD, Davies MJ. Sleep disturbances in women with polycystic ovary syndrome: Prevalence, pathophysiology, impact and management strategies. Nat Sci Sleep. 2018 Feb 1;10:45–64. doi: 10.2147/NSS.S127475. PMID: 29440941; PMCID: PMC5799701.

31. Fogel RB, Malhotra A, Pillar G, Pittman SD, Dunaif A, White DP. Increased prevalence of obstructive sleep apnea syndrome in obese women with polycystic ovary syndrome. J Clin Endocrinol Metab. 2001 Mar;86(3):1175–1180. doi: 10.1210/jcem.86.3.7316. PMID: 11238505.

32. Vgontzas AN, Legro RS, Bixler EO, Grayev A, Kales A, Chrousos GP. Polycystic ovary syndrome is associated with obstructive sleep apnea and daytime sleepiness: Role of insulin resistance. J Clin Endocrinol Metab. 2001 Feb;86(2):517–520. doi: 10.1210/jcem.86.2.7185. PMID: 11158002.

33. Doycheva I, Ehrmann DA. Nonalcoholic fatty liver disease and obstructive sleep apnea in women with polycystic ovary syndrome. Fertil Steril. 2022 May;117(5):897–911. doi: 10.1016/j.fertnstert.2022.03.020. PMID: 35512974.

34. Teede HJ, Misso ML, Costello MF, Dokras A, Laven J, Moran L, Piltonen T, Norman RJ; International PCOS Network. Recommendations from the international evidence-based guideline for the assessment and management of polycystic ovary syndrome. Fertil Steril. 2018 Aug;110(3):364–379. doi: 10.1016/j.fertnstert.2018.05.004. Epub 2018 Jul 19. PMID: 30033227; PMCID: PMC6939856/.

35. Kohn TP, Kohn JR, Haney NM, Pastuszak AW, Lipshultz LI. The effect of sleep on men's health. Transl Androl Urol. 2020 Mar;9(Suppl 2):S178–S185. doi: 10.21037/tau.2019.11.07. PMID: 32257858; PMCID: PMC7108988.

36. Freeman JR, Whitcomb BW, Bertone-Johnson ER, Balzer LB, O'Brien LM, Dunietz GL, Purdue-Smithe AC, Kim K, Silver RM, Schisterman EF, Mumford SL. Preconception sleep duration, sleep timing, and shift work in association with fecundability and live birth among women with a history of pregnancy loss. Fertil Steril. 2023 Feb;119(2):252–263. doi: 10.1016/j.fertnstert.2022.10.026. Epub 2022 Dec 29. PMID: 36586812.

37. Caetano G, Bozinovic I, Dupont C, Léger D, Lévy R, Sermondade N. Impact of sleep on female and male reproductive functions: A systematic review. Fertil Steril. 2021 Mar;115(3):715–731. doi:10.1016/j.fertnstert.2020.08.1429. Epub 2020 Oct 11. PMID: 33054981.

38. Lin JL, Lin YH, Chueh KH. Somatic symptoms, psychological distress, and sleep disturbance among infertile women with intrauterine insemination treatment. J Clin Nurs. 2014 Jun;23(11–12):1677–1684. doi: 10.1111/jocn.12306. Epub 2013 Jul 5. PMID: 23829562.

39. Kirca N, Ongen M. Perceived stress and sleep quality before oocyte pick-up, embryo transfer, and pregnancy test in women receiving in vitro fertilization treatment. Sleep Breath. 2021 Dec;25(4):1977–1985. doi: 10.1007/s11325-021-02328-w. Epub 2021 Feb 23. PMID: 33624218.

40. Goldstein CA, Lanham MS, Smith YR, O'Brien LM. Sleep in women undergoing in vitro fertilization: A pilot study. Sleep Med. 2017 Apr;32:105–113. doi: 10.1016/j.sleep.2016.12.007. Epub 2016 Dec 21. PMID: 28366321; PMCID: PMC5380145.

41. Faraut B, Bayon V, Léger D. Neuroendocrine, immune and oxidative stress in shift workers. Sleep Med Rev. 2013 Dec;17(6):433–444. doi: 10.1016/j.smrv.2012.12.006. Epub 2013 Apr 22. PMID: 23618533.

42. Liu Z, Zheng Y, Wang B, Li J, Qin L, Li X, Liu X, Bian Y, Chen Z, Zhao H, Zhao S. The impact of sleep on in vitro fertilization embryo transfer outcomes: A prospective study. Fertil Steril. 2023 Jan;119(1):47–55. doi: 10.1016/j.fertnstert.2022.10.015. Epub 2022 Nov 23. PMID: 36435629.

43. Kervezee L, Shechter A, Boivin DB. Impact of shift work on the circadian timing system and health in women. Sleep Med Clin. 2018 Sep;13(3):295–306. doi: 10.1016/j.jsmc.2018.04.003. PMID: 30098749.

44. Mahoney MM. Shift work, jet lag, and female reproduction. Int J Endocrinol. 2010;2010:813764. doi: 10.1155/2010/813764. Epub 2010 Mar 8. PMID: 20224815; PMCID: PMC2834958.

45. Bisanti L, Olsen J, Basso O, Thonneau P, Karmaus W. Shift work and subfecundity: a European multicenter study. European Study Group on Infertility and Subfecundity. J Occup Environ Med. 1996 Apr;38(4):352–358. doi: 10.1097/00043764-199604000-00012. PMID: 8925318.

46. Fernandez RC, Moore VM, Marino JL, Whitrow MJ, Davies MJ. Night shift among women: Is it associated with difficulty conceiving a first birth? Front Public Health. 2020 Dec 1;8:595943. doi: 10.3389/fpubh.2020.595943. PMID: 33335878; PMCID: PMC7736040.

47. Fernandez RC, Marino JL, Varcoe TJ, Davis S, Moran LJ, Rumbold AR, Brown HM, Whitrow MJ, Davies MJ, Moore VM. Fixed or rotating night shift work undertaken by women: Implications for fertility and miscarriage. Semin Reprod Med. 2016 Mar;34(2):74–82. doi: 10.1055/s-0036 -1571354. Epub 2016 Feb 8. PMID: 26854708.

48. Gamble KL, Resuehr D, Johnson CH. Shift work and circadian dysregulation of reproduction. Front Endocrinol (Lausanne). 2013 Aug 7;4:92. doi: 10.3389/fendo.2013.00092. PMID: 23966978; PMCID: PMC3736045.

49. Cai C, Vandermeer B, Khurana R, Nerenberg K, Featherstone R, Sebastianski M, Davenport MH. The impact of occupational shift work and working hours during pregnancy on health outcomes: a systematic review and meta-analysis. Am J Obstet Gynecol. 2019 Dec;221(6):563–576. doi: 10.1016/j.ajog.2019.06.051. Epub 2019 Jul 2. PMID: 31276631.

Chapter 12 References

1. Malik VS, Hu FB. The role of sugar-sweetened beverages in the global epidemics of obesity and chronic diseases. Nat Rev Endocrinol. 2022 Apr;18(4):205–218. doi: 10.1038/s41574-021-00627 -6. Epub 2022 Jan 21. PMID: 35064240; PMCID: PMC8778490.

2. Fowler SP, Williams K, Resendez RG, Hunt KJ, Hazuda HP, Stern MP. Fueling the obesity epidemic? Artificially sweetened beverage use and long-term weight gain. Obesity (Silver Spring). 2008 Aug;16(8):1894–1900. doi: 10.1038/oby.2008.284. Epub 2008 Jun 5. PMID: 18535548.

3. Cleveland Clinic. This is why artificial sweeteners are bad for you. health.clevelandclinic.org /whats-worse-sugar-or-artificial-sweetener/. Accessed 9/26/23.

4. Riboli E, Beland FA, Lachenmeier DW, Marques MM, Phillips DH, Schernhammer E, Afghan A, Assunção R, Caderni G, Corton JC, de Aragão Umbuzeiro G, de Jong D, Deschasaux-Tanguy M, Hodge A, Ishihara J, Levy DD, Mandrioli D, McCullough ML, McNaughton SA, Morita T, Nugent AP, Ogawa K, Pandiri AR, Sergi CM, Touvier M, Zhang L, Benbrahim-Tallaa L, Chittiboyina S, Cuomo D, DeBono NL, Debras C, de Conti A, El Ghissassi F, Fontvieille E, Harewood R, Kaldor J, Mattock H, Pasqual E, Rigutto G, Simba H, Suonio E, Viegas S, Wedekind R, Schubauer-Berigan MK, Madia F. Carcinogenicity of aspartame, methyleugenol, and isoeugenol. Lancet Oncol. 2023 Jul 13:S1470–2045(23)00341-8. doi: 10.1016/S1470-2045(23)00341-8. Epub ahead of print. PMID: 37454664.

5. Cho NA, Klancic T, Nettleton JE, Paul HA, Reimer RA. Impact of food ingredients (aspartame, sttevia, prebiotic oligofructose) on fertility and reproductive outcomes in obese rats. Obesity (Silver Spring). 2018 Nov;26(11):1692–1695. doi: 10.1002/oby.22325. PMID: 30358146.

6. Calleja-Conde J, Echeverry-Alzate V, Bühler KM, Durán-González P, Morales-García JÁ, Segovia-Rodríguez L, Rodríguez de Fonseca F, Giné E, López-Moreno JA. The immune system through the lens of alcohol intake and gut microbiota. Int J Mol Sci. 2021 Jul 13;22(14):7485. doi: 10.3390 /ijms22147485. PMID: 34299105; PMCID: PMC8303153.

7. Freudenheim JL. Alcohol's effects on breast cancer in women. Alcohol Res. 2020 Jun 18;40(2):11. doi: 10.35946/arcr.v40.2.11. PMID: 32582503; PMCID: PMC7295577.

8. Rossi BV, Berry KF, Hornstein MD, Cramer DW, Ehrlich S, Missmer SA. Effect of alcohol consumption on in vitro fertilization. Obstet Gynecol. 2011 Jan;117(1):136–142. doi: 10.1097/AOG.0b013e31820090e1. PMID: 21173655; PMCID: PMC4487775.

9. Nicolau P, Miralpeix E, Solà I, Carreras R, Checa MA. Alcohol consumption and in vitro fertilization: a review of the literature. Gynecol Endocrinol. 2014 Nov;30(11):759–763. doi: 10.3109/09513590.2014.938623. Epub 2014 Jul 9. PMID: 25007008.

10. Rao W, Li Y, Li N, Yao Q, Li Y. The association between caffeine and alcohol consumption and IVF/ICSI outcomes: A systematic review and dose-response meta-analysis. Acta Obstet Gynecol Scand. 2022 Oct 19. doi: 10.1111/aogs.14464. Epub ahead of print. PMID: 36259227.

11. Klonoff-Cohen H, Lam-Kruglick P, Gonzalez C. Effects of maternal and paternal alcohol consumption on the success rates of in vitro fertilization and gamete intrafallopian transfer. Fertil Steril. 2003 Feb;79(2):330–339. doi: 10.1016/s0015-0282(02)04582-x. PMID: 12568842.

12. Fan D, Liu L, Xia Q, Wang W, Wu S, Tian G, Liu Y, Ni J, Wu S, Guo X, Liu Z. Female alcohol consumption and fecundability: A systematic review and dose-response meta-analysis. Sci Rep. 2017 Oct 23;7(1):13815. doi: 10.1038/s41598-017-14261-8. PMID: 29062133; PMCID: PMC5653745.

13. Anwar MY, Marcus M, Taylor KC. The association between alcohol intake and fecundability during menstrual cycle phases. Hum Reprod. 2021 Aug 18;36(9):2538–2548. doi: 10.1093/humrep/deab121. PMID: 34102671; PMCID: PMC8561243.

14. Asiedu B, Nyakudya TT, Lembede BW, Chivandi E. Early-life exposure to alcohol and the risk of alcohol-induced liver disease in adulthood. Birth Defects Res. 2021 Apr 1;113(6):451–468. doi: 10.1002/bdr2.1881. Epub 2021 Feb 12. PMID: 33577143.

15. Gupta KK, Gupta VK, Shirasaka T. An update on fetal alcohol syndrome-pathogenesis, risks, and treatment. Alcohol Clin Exp Res. 2016 Aug;40(8):1594–1602. doi: 10.1111/acer.13135. Epub 2016 Jul 4. PMID: 27375266.

16. Practice Committee of the American Society for Reproductive Medicine. Electronic address: asrm@asrm.org; Practice Committee of the American Society for Reproductive Medicine. Smoking and infertility: A committee opinion. Fertil Steril. 2018 Sep;110(4):611–618. doi: 10.1016/j.fertnstert.2018.06.016. PMID: 30196946.

17. Waylen AL, Metwally M, Jones GL, Wilkinson AJ, Ledger WL. Effects of cigarette smoking upon clinical outcomes of assisted reproduction: A meta-analysis. Hum Reprod Update. 2009 Jan-Feb;15(1):31–44. doi: 10.1093/humupd/dmn046. Epub 2008 Oct 15. PMID: 18927070.

18. Källén K. The impact of maternal smoking during pregnancy on delivery outcome. Eur J Public Health. 2001 Sep;11(3):329–333. doi: 10.1093/eurpub/11.3.329. PMID: 11582615.

19. Kleckner AS, Kleckner IR, Kamen CS, Tejani MA, Janelsins MC, Morrow GR, Peppone LJ. Opportunities for cannabis in supportive care in cancer. Ther Adv Med Oncol. 2019 Aug 1;11:1758835919866362. doi: 10.1177/1758835919866362. PMID: 31413731; PMCID: PMC6676264.

20. Abrams DI, Guzman M. Cannabis in cancer care. Clin Pharmacol Ther. 2015 Jun;97(6):575–586. doi: 10.1002/cpt.108. Epub 2015 Apr 17. PMID: 25777363.10.1177/1758835919866362. PMID: 31413731; PMCID: PMC6676264.

21. Volkow ND, Baler RD, Compton WM, Weiss SR. Adverse health effects of marijuana use. N Engl J Med. 2014 Jun 5;370(23):2219–2227. doi: 10.1056/NEJMra1402309. PMID: 24897085; PMCID: PMC4827335.

22. Ford TC, Hayley AC, Downey LA, Parrott AC. Cannabis: An overview of its adverse acute and chronic effects and its implications. Curr Drug Abuse Rev. 2017;10(1):6–18. doi: 10.2174 / 1874473710666170712113042. PMID: 28707583.

23. Gurney J, Shaw C, Stanley J, Signal V, Sarfati D. Cannabis exposure and risk of testicular cancer: a systematic review and meta-analysis. BMC Cancer. 2015 Nov 11;15:897. doi: 10.1186/s12885-015 -1905-6. PMID: 26560314; PMCID: PMC4642772.

24. Fonseca BM, Rebelo I. Cannabis and cannabinoids in reproduction and fertility: Where we stand. Reprod Sci. 2022 Sep;29(9):2429–2439. doi: 10.1007/s43032-021-00588-1. Epub 2021 May 10. PMID: 33970442.

25. Badowski S, Smith G. Cannabis use during pregnancy and postpartum. Can Fam Physician. 2020 Feb;66(2):98–103. PMID: 32060189; PMCID: PMC7021337.

26. Lo JO, Hedges JC, Girardi G. Impact of cannabinoids on pregnancy, reproductive health, and off-spring outcomes. Am J Obstet Gynecol. 2022 Oct;227(4):571–581. doi: 10.1016/j.ajog.2022.05.056. Epub 2022 May 31. PMID: 35662548; PMCID: PMC9530020.

27. Ilnitsky S, Van Uum S. Marijuana and fertility. CMAJ. 2019 Jun 10;191(23):E638. doi: 10.1503 /cmaj.181577. PMID: 31182459; PMCID: PMC6565391.

28. Fonseca BM, Rebelo I. Cannabis and cannabinoids in reproduction and fertility: Where we stand. Reprod Sci. 2022 Sep;29(9):2429–2439. doi: 10.1007/s43032-021-00588-1. Epub 2021 May 10. PMID: 33970442.

29. Misner MJ, Taborek A, Dufour J, Sharifi L, Khokhar JY, Favetta LA. Effects of delta-9 tetrahydro-cannabinol (THC) on oocyte competence and early embryonic development. Front Toxicol. 2021 Mar 23;3:647918. doi: 10.3389/ftox.2021.647918. PMID: 35295104; PMCID: PMC8915882.

30. Fuchs Weizman N, Wyse BA, Montbriand J, Jahangiri S, Librach CL. Cannabis significantly alters DNA methylation of the human ovarian follicle in a concentration-dependent manner. Mol Hum Reprod. 2022 Jun 8;28(7):gaac022. doi: 10.1093/molehr/gaac022. Epub ahead of print. PMID: 35674367; PMCID: PMC9247704.

31. Schrott R, Murphy SK. Cannabis use and the sperm epigenome: a budding concern? Environ Epigenet. 2020 Mar 19;6(1):dvaa002. doi: 10.1093/eep/dvaa002. PMID: 32211199; PMCID: PMC7081939.

32. Pizzol D, Demurtas J, Stubbs B, Soysal P, Mason C, Isik AT, Solmi M, Smith L, Veronese N. Relationship between cannabis use and erectile dysfunction: A systematic review and meta-analysis. Am J Mens Health. 2019 Nov-Dec;13(6):1557988319892464. doi: 10.1177/1557988319892464. PMID: 31795801; PMCID: PMC6893937.

33. Hehemann MC, Raheem OA, Rajanahally S, Holt S, Chen T, Fustok JN, Song K, Rylander H, Chow E, Ostrowski KA, Muller CH, Walsh TJ. Evaluation of the impact of marijuana use on semen quality: A prospective analysis. Ther Adv Urol. 2021 Jul 20;13:17562872211032484. doi: 10.1177/17562872211032484. PMID: 34367341; PMCID: PMC8299873.

34. Gundersen TD, Jørgensen N, Andersson AM, Bang AK, Nordkap L, Skakkebæk NE, Priskorn L, Juul A, Jensen TK. Association between use of marijuana and male reproductive hormones and semen quality: A study among 1,215 healthy young men. Am J Epidemiol. 2015 Sep 15;182(6):473–481. doi: 10.1093/aje/kwv135. Epub 2015 Aug 16. PMID: 26283092.

35. Wise LA, Wesselink AK, Hatch EE, Rothman KJ, Mikkelsen EM, Sørensen HT, Mahalingaiah S. Marijuana use and fecundability in a North American preconception cohort study. J Epidemiol Community Health. 2018 Mar;72(3):208–215. doi: 10.1136/jech-2017-209755. Epub 2017 Dec 22. PMID: 29273628.

36. Kasman AM, Thoma ME, McLain AC, Eisenberg ML. Association between use of marijuana and time to pregnancy in men and women: findings from the National Survey of Family Growth. Fertil Steril. 2018 May;109(5):866–871. doi: 10.1016/j.fertnstert.2018.01.015. Epub 2018 Mar 16. PMID: 29555335.

37. Mumford SL, Flannagan KS, Radoc JG, Sjaarda LA, Zolton JR, Metz TD, Plowden TC, Perkins NJ, DeVilbiss EA, Andriessen VC, Purdue-Smithe AC, Kim K, Yisahak SF, Freeman JR, Alkhalaf Z, Silver RM, Schisterman EF. Cannabis use while trying to conceive: a prospective cohort study evaluating associations with fecundability, live birth and pregnancy loss. Hum Reprod. 2021 Apr 20;36(5):1405–1415. doi: 10.1093/humrep/deaa355. PMID: 33421071; PMCID: PMC8679412.

38. Mumford SL, Flannagan KS, Radoc JG, Sjaarda LA, Zolton JR, Metz TD, Plowden TC, Perkins NJ, DeVilbiss EA, Andriessen VC, Purdue-Smithe AC, Kim K, Yisahak SF, Freeman JR, Alkhalaf Z, Silver RM, Schisterman EF. Cannabis use while trying to conceive: a prospective cohort study evaluating associations with fecundability, live birth and pregnancy loss. Hum Reprod. 2021 Apr 20;36(5):1405–1415. doi: 10.1093/humrep/deaa355. PMID: 33421071; PMCID: PMC8679412.

39. Ricci E, Viganò P, Cipriani S, Somigliana E, Chiaffarino F, Bulfoni A, Parazzini F. Coffee and caffeine intake and male infertility: A systematic review. Nutr J. 2017 Jun 24;16(1):37. doi: 10.1186/s12937-017-0257-2. PMID: 28646871; PMCID: PMC5482951.

40. Karmon AE, Toth TL, Chiu YH, Gaskins AJ, Tanrikut C, Wright DL, Hauser R, Chavarro JE; Earth Study Team. Male caffeine and alcohol intake in relation to semen parameters and in vitro fertilization outcomes among fertility patients. Andrology. 2017 Mar;5(2):354–361. doi: 10.1111/andr.12310. Epub 2017 Feb 10. PMID: 28187518; PMCID: PMC5352521.

41. Gaskins AJ, Chavarro JE. Diet and fertility: A review. Am J Obstet Gynecol. 2018 Apr;218(4):379–389. doi: 10.1016/j.ajog.2017.08.010. Epub 2017 Aug 24. PMID: 28844822; PMCID: PMC5826784.

42. Purdue-Smithe AC, Kim K, Schliep KC, DeVilbiss EA, Hinkle SN, Ye A, Perkins NJ, Sjaarda LA, Silver RM, Schisterman EF, Mumford SL. Preconception caffeine metabolites, caffeinated beverage intake, and fecundability. Am J Clin Nutr. 2022 Apr 1;115(4):1227–1236. doi: 10.1093/ajcn/nqab435. PMID: 35030239; PMCID: PMC8970989.

43. Machtinger R, Gaskins AJ, Mansur A, Adir M, Racowsky C, Baccarelli AA, Hauser R, Chavarro JE. Association between preconception maternal beverage intake and in vitro fertilization outcomes. Fertil Steril. 2017 Dec;108(6):1026–1033. doi: 10.1016/j.fertnstert.2017.09.007. Epub 2017 Oct 3. PMID: 28985907; PMCID: PMC5716855.

44. Lyngsø J, Kesmodel US, Bay B, Ingerslev HJ, Nybo Andersen AM, Ramlau-Hansen CH. Impact of female daily coffee consumption on successful fertility treatment: A Danish cohort study. Fertil Steril. 2019 Jul;112(1):120–129.e2. doi: 10.1016/j.fertnstert.2019.03.014. Epub 2019 Apr 28. PMID: 31043232.

45. Rao W, Li Y, Li N, Yao Q, Li Y. The association between caffeine and alcohol consumption and IVF/ICSI outcomes: A systematic review and dose-response meta-analysis. Acta Obstet Gynecol Scand. 2022 Oct 19. doi: 10.1111/aogs.14464. Epub ahead of print. PMID: 36259227.

46. Greenwood DC, Thatcher NJ, Ye J, Garrard L, Keogh G, King LG, Cade JE. Caffeine intake during pregnancy and adverse birth outcomes: A systematic review and dose-response meta-analysis. Eur J Epidemiol. 2014 Oct;29(10):725–734. doi: 10.1007/s10654-014-9944-x. Epub 2014 Sep 2. PMID: 25179792.

47. Gaskins AJ, Rich-Edwards JW, Williams PL, Toth TL, Missmer SA, Chavarro JE. Pre-pregnancy caffeine and caffeinated beverage intake and risk of spontaneous abortion. Eur J Nutr. 2018 Feb;57(1):107–117. doi: 10.1007/s00394-016-1301-2. Epub 2016 Aug 29. PMID: 27573467; PMCID: PMC5332346.

48. Darbre, PD. Chemical components of plastics as endocrine disruptors: Overview and commentary. Birth Defects Research. 2020; 112: 1300–1307. https://doi.org/10.1002/bdr2.1778.

49. Rochester JR. Bisphenol A and human health: A review of the literature. Reprod Toxicol. 2013 Dec;42:132–155. doi: 10.1016/j.reprotox.2013.08.008. Epub 2013 Aug 30. PMID: 23994667.

50. Eladak S, Grisin T, Moison D, Guerquin MJ, N'Tumba-Byn T, Pozzi-Gaudin S, Benachi A, Livera G, Rouiller-Fabre V, Habert R. A new chapter in the bisphenol A story: Bisphenol S and bisphenol F are not safe alternatives to this compound. Fertil Steril. 2015 Jan;103(1):11–21. doi: 10.1016/j .fertnstert.2014.11.005. Epub 2014 Dec 2. PMID: 25475787.

51. Allen, Joseph. Opinion: Stop playing whack-a-mole with hazardous chemicals. Washington Post, December 15, 2016. www.washingtonpost.com/opinions/stop-playing-whack-a-mole-with -hazardous-chemicals/.

52. Blackburn, B., Cox, K., Zhang, Y., Anderson, D., Wilkins, D., & Porucznik, C. (2020). Effect of rinsing canned foods on bisphenol-A exposure: The hummus experiment. *Experimental Results, 1*, E45. doi:10.1017/exp.2020.52.

53. Panagiotou EM, Ojasalo V, Damdimopoulou P. Phthalates, ovarian function and fertility in adulthood. Best Pract Res Clin Endocrinol Metab. 2021 Sep;35(5):101552. doi: 10.1016/j .beem.2021.101552. Epub 2021 Jun 2. PMID: 34238683.

54. Oluwayiose OA, Marcho C, Wu H, Houle E, Krawetz SA, Suvorov A, Mager J, Richard Pilsner J. Paternal preconception phthalate exposure alters sperm methylome and embryonic programming. Environ Int. 2021 Oct;155:106693. doi: 10.1016/j.envint.2021.106693. Epub 2021 Jun 10. PMID: 34120004; PMCID: PMC8292217.

55. Arya S, Dwivedi AK, Alvarado L, Kupesic-Plavsic Ṣ. Exposure of U.S. population to endocrine disruptive chemicals (parabens, benzophenone-3, bisphenol-A and triclosan) and their associations with female infertility. Environ Pollut. 2020 Oct;265(Pt A):114763. doi: 10.1016/j.envpol.2020.114763. Epub 2020 May 8. PMID: 32806428.

56. Karwacka A, Zamkowska D, Radwan M, Jurewicz J. Exposure to modern, widespread environmental endocrine disrupting chemicals and their effect on the reproductive potential of women: An overview of current epidemiological evidence. Hum Fertil (Camb). 2019 Apr;22(1):2–25. doi: 10.1080/14647273.2017.1358828. Epub 2017 Jul 31. PMID: 28758506.

57. J. Allen, "These Toxic Chemicals Are Everywhere—Even in Your Body. And They Won't Ever Go Away," Washington Post, January 2, 2018.

58. Kim YR, White N, Bräunig J, Vijayasarathy S, Mueller JF, Knox CL, Harden FA, Pacella R, Toms LL. Per- and poly-fluoroalkyl substances (PFASs) in follicular fluid from women experiencing infertility in Australia. Environ Res. 2020 Nov;190:109963. doi: 10.1016/j.envres.2020.109963. Epub 2020 Jul 21. PMID: 32745751.

59. Hong A, Zhuang L, Cui W, Lu Q, Yang P, Su S, Wang B, Zhang G, Chen D. Per- and polyfluoroalkyl substances (PFAS) exposure in women seeking in vitro fertilization-embryo transfer treatment (IVF-ET) in China: Blood-follicular transfer and associations with IVF-ET outcomes. Sci Total Environ. 2022 Sep 10;838(Pt 3):156323. doi: 10.1016/j.scitotenv.2022.156323. Epub 2022 May 28. PMID: 35636536.

60. Karwacka A, Zamkowska D, Radwan M, Jurewicz J. Exposure to modern, widespread environmental endocrine disrupting chemicals and their effect on the reproductive potential of women: An overview of current epidemiological evidence. Hum Fertil (Camb). 2019 Apr;22(1):2–25. doi: 10.1080/14647273.2017.1358828. Epub 2017 Jul 31. PMID: 28758506.

61. Blackburn K, Green D. The potential effects of microplastics on human health: What is known and what is unknown. Ambio. 2022 Mar;51(3):518–530. doi: 10.1007/s13280-021-01589-9. Epub 2021 Jun 29. PMID: 34185251; PMCID: PMC8800959.

62. D'Angelo S, Meccariello R. Microplastics: A threat for male fertility. Int J Environ Res Public Health. 2021 Mar 1;18(5):2392. doi: 10.3390/ijerph18052392. PMID: 33804513; PMCID: PMC7967748.

63. Zhang C, Chen J, Ma S, Sun Z, Wang Z. Microplastics may be a significant cause of male infertility. Am J Mens Health. 2022 May-Jun;16(3):15579883221096549. doi: 10.1177/15579883221096549. PMID: 35608037; PMCID: PMC9134445.

64. Wei Z, Wang Y, Wang S, Xie J, Han Q, Chen M. Comparing the effects of polystyrene microplastics exposure on reproduction and fertility in male and female mice. Toxicology. 2022 Jan 15;465:153059. doi: 10.1016/j.tox.2021.153059. Epub 2021 Dec 2. PMID: 34864092.

65. Canipari R, De Santis L, Cecconi S. Female fertility and environmental pollution. Int J Environ Res Public Health. 2020 Nov 26;17(23):8802. doi: 10.3390/ijerph17238802. PMID: 33256215; PMCID: PMC7730072.

66. Lin Y, Zou J, Yang W, Li CQ. A review of recent advances in research on PM2.5 in China. Int J Environ Res Public Health. 2018 Mar 2;15(3):438. doi: 10.3390/ijerph15030438. PMID: 29498704; PMCID: PMC5876983.

67. Carré J, Gatimel N, Moreau J, Parinaud J, Léandri R. Does air pollution play a role in infertility?: a systematic review. Environ Health. 2017 Jul 28;16(1):82. doi: 10.1186/s12940-017-0291-8. PMID: 28754128; PMCID: PMC5534122.

68. Conforti A, Mascia M, Cioffi G, De Angelis C, Coppola G, De Rosa P, Pivonello R, Alviggi C, De Placido G. Air pollution and female fertility: A systematic review of literature. Reprod Biol Endocrinol. 2018 Dec 30;16(1):117. doi: 10.1186/s12958-018-0433-z. PMID: 30594197; PMCID: PMC6311303.

69. Checa Vizcaíno MA, González-Comadran M, Jacquemin B. Outdoor air pollution and human infertility: A systematic review. Fertil Steril. 2016 Sep 15;106(4):897–904.e1. doi: 10.1016/j.fertnstert.2016.07.1110. Epub 2016 Aug 8. PMID: 27513553.

70. Gaskins AJ, Mínguez-Alarcón L, Fong KC, Abdelmessih S, Coull BA, Chavarro JE, Schwartz J, Kloog I, Souter I, Hauser R, Laden F. Exposure to fine particulate matter and ovarian reserve among women from a fertility clinic. Epidemiology. 2019 Jul;30(4):486–491. doi: 10.1097/EDE.0000000000001029. PMID: 31162281; PMCID: PMC6550330.

71. Knapke ET, Magalhaes DP, Dalvie MA, Mandrioli D, Perry MJ. Environmental and occupational pesticide exposure and human sperm parameters: A Navigation Guide review. Toxicology. 2022 Jan 15;465:153017. doi: 10.1016/j.tox.2021.153017. Epub 2021 Oct 29. PMID: 34756984.

72. Ingaramo P, Alarcón R, Muñoz-de-Toro M, Luque EH. Are glyphosate and glyphosate-based herbicides endocrine disruptors that alter female fertility? Mol Cell Endocrinol. 2020 Dec 1;518:110934. doi: 10.1016/j.mce.2020.110934. Epub 2020 Jul 10. PMID: 32659439.

Index

beans, 24, 55, 85n*, 93, 121, 175–176, 207

beef, 125. *see also* red meat

beets, 43

beta-carotene, 44–45

betalain, 43

beverages, sugary, 6, 17, 198–200, 205

binge eating, 186n**

bisphenols, 206–208, 233

blood sugar, 72, 87, 198

blueberries, 46

blue fruit and vegetables, 45–46, 223

box breathing, 189

bran, 69, 71

Brazil nuts, 153, 154

breast cancer, 87–88, 201

breath work, 186n*, 189

broccoli, 144–145

budget-friendly cooking, 93, 123

B vitamins, 47, 48, 66, 69, 87, 105, 109, 118,
153

C

cabbage, 97–98

caffeine, 189n**, 190, 204–206

calcium, 38, 41, 103–105, 108, 109, 153

cancer, 87–88, 118, 124, 126, 165, 201

cannabidiol (CBD), 203

cannabis, 203–204, 233

canola oil, 155–156

carbohydrates, 36, 65n**, 71–73, 110, 117, 217

cardiovascular conditioning, 179n**, 184

cardiovascular disease, 38, 118, 126, 141, 151,
165

carotenoids, 39, 42, 44, 153

cashew milk, 109

celiac disease, 65n*, 67–68

certified humane eggs, 122

Chavarro, Jorge E., 10–11

cheese, 56, 103, 104

chia seeds, 143, 158, 160

chickpeas, 91

cholesterol, 150

choline, 38, 118, 120, 121, 123–124, 136, 169,
173

citrus fruit, 44

clean eating, 2, 193–195

coconut products, 109, 110, 150, 156

cod, 140

coenzyme A, 48

coenzyme Q10, 17, 168, 171–172, 174

comfort food, 52

complex carbohydrates, 36, 71, 72

confidence, xiii, 24–26, 28, 147

convenience foods, 2, 81–82

conventionally-grown produce, 49–50, 207

cooking, 165, 197n*
  batch, 73–74
  budget-friendly, 93, 123
  fats in, 154–156
  and fertility blueprint, 216–217
  fish, 140–141
  legumes, 90–93
  and meal planning, 141
  mushrooms, 52
  oats, 74
  proteins, 124
  sugar/sweeteners in, 200
  vegetables, 50–52
  whole grains, 73

copper, 47, 66, 87, 153

cruciferous vegetables, 41–42, 218, 219, 222

culinary medicine, 27–28

cyanocobalamin, 128

D

dairy products, 103–115, 121
  calcium in, 105
  fertility benefits of, 105–106
  on Fertility Plate, 22–24
  health benefits of, 105

vitamin D, 12, 47, 67, 74, 105–109, 120, 122, 136, 140, 151, 168, 170, 171, 174
vitamin E, 39, 66, 108, 151, 153
vitamin K, 41, 45, 104, 108, 122, 151

W

walking, 184, 185, 218–222, 232
weight loss, 7–8, 26, 87, 161–162
wheat, 67, 68
white beans, 146, 218
white fish, 139, 142
white fruit and vegetables, 46–47

whole foods, 29, 200
whole grains. *see* grains, whole
Willett, Walter C., 10–11

Y

yellow fruit and vegetables, 44–45, 222
yogurt, 92, 104, 106, 110–111
Yogurt Fruit Parfait (recipe), 111

Z

zeaxanthin, 44
zinc, 47, 48, 66, 74, 75, 87, 118, 136, 153, 169, 173

About the Authors

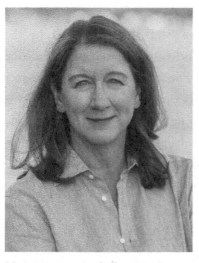

Angela Thyer, MD, is a board-certified physician in reproductive endocrinology and infertility, and obstetrics and gynecology, and is a diplomate of the American College of Lifestyle Medicine. She's a graduate of Duke University and the University of Cincinnati College of Medicine. Angela completed her residency at Oregon Health & Science University and her fellowship in reproductive endocrinology and infertility at the University of Texas at San Antonio. Her interests include nutrition, exercise, fertility, lifestyle medicine, healthy aging, and polycystic ovary syndrome (PCOS). She served on the faculty at the University of Washington and in 2004 cofounded Seattle Reproductive Medicine (SRM), the largest fertility practice on the West Coast. She went on to develop the Food for Fertility program with Judy Simon in 2012.

Angela holds leadership roles in the American Society of Reproductive Medicine Nutritional Special Interest Group and the American College of Lifestyle Medicine Reproductive subcommittee of the Women's Health Member Interest Group. She is a certified plant-based chef through Rouxbe and is passionate about sharing recipes and cooking techniques with everyone. She lives in Seattle, Washington, with her husband and enjoys visiting her two daughters on both coasts.

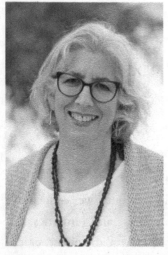

Judy Simon, RDN, is a registered dietitian nutritionist who specializes in reproductive health. She is the founder of Mind Body Nutrition, LLC, and a clinical instructor and staff dietitian at the University of Washington. Judy's expertise includes polycystic ovary syndrome (PCOS), fertility, eating disorders, weight inclusive care, culinary medicine, and reproductive health.

Judy has held leadership roles in the American Society of Reproductive Medicine Nutritional Special Interest Group and is a Fellow of the Academy of Nutrition and Dietetics.

Judy's inclusive approach to health is to meet people where they are. She helps them find small changes in their daily habits, which can inch them toward better health. Integrating mindfulness, planning, and accountability, all while taking a nonjudgmental, down-to-earth approach, allows Judy to help many women have healthier, more fertile lives.